Praise for *The Comp...* KT-549-625

'Th...
an...
bal... ...and the v...
cou... ...nd specialists alike. I have no dou...
abo... embark on or already going through...
wil... in this book a useful companion at every...
the v...

Tare... -Toukhy, Consultant in Reproductive Medicine,
Guy... id St Thomas' Hospital

'As th... .tle of the book says, this really is a *complete* guide to
IVF fr... ı what the waiting room might look like right through
to pre... ıplantation diagnosis and complementary therapies.
Kate ... ın asks all the questions that we at Infertility Network
UK ... asked, including some that some patients might be
nervc... about asking their clinician. Best of all, the questions
are a... ʒered clearly, sympathetically and honestly.'
Clar... ewis-Jones, Chief Executive Infertility Network
UK ... l More to Life

'A ... horitative book which combines factual accuracy with
i ... ve understanding of how couples deal with the complexi-
... IVF treatment.'
ssor Siladitya Bhattacharya, Professor of
ductive Medicine, Head, Section of Applied
al Sciences, University of Aberdeen, Aberdeen
nity Hospital

...ate Brian has done it again. Straightforward information and
ʒuidance from someone who knows her way round the fertility
industry and has been through the pain and confusion of difficulties with conception and the rollercoaster of IVF herself.
Writing, as always, with refreshing simplicity and candour,
Kate detail... ...bers of

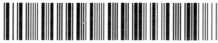

individuals and couples are now making when creating a family without help is no longer an option. From what to expect in a fertility clinic waiting room to the intricacies of testicular biopsies, via counselling and the importance of telling donor conceived children about their origins, this lovely book will inform, guide and reassure all men and women, single women and lesbian couples needing IVF procedures.'

Olivia Montuschi, Donor Conception Network

'The amount of information available to couples seeking advice about fertility treatment is now vast, yet the complexity of IVF and the desire of couples to understand its intricacies remain. As a scientist who has worked within this field for over twenty years I am all too aware of how difficult it sometimes is to convey to couples details about the medical and biological processes that comprise their treatment – this is where Kate has excelled. Not only has she managed to describe highly complex processes in a manner that is very easily understandable, her writing style is such that one is constantly enticed to read on.

The factual accuracy and personal experience described within the pages of this book are a testament to the extensive research that Kate has undertaken – if all our patients had read this book a lot of their anxieties and uncertainties would most certainly have gone away.'

Dr Stephen Troup, Chair, Association of Clinical Embryologists

The complete guide to

IVF

An Insider's Guide to Fertility Clinics and Treatments

KATE BRIAN

PIATKUS

PIATKUS

First published in Great Britain in 2009 by Piatkus Books

Copyright © 2009 by Kate Brian

The moral right of the author has been asserted

A CIP catalogue record for this book
is available from the British Library

ISBN 978-0-7499-0970-3

Edited by Jan Cutler
Medical advice from Tarek El-Toukhy, Consultant in Reproductive Medicine, Guy's and
St. Thomas' Hospital
Typeset in ITC Esprit by Palimpsest Book Production Limited, Grangemouth, Stirlingshire
Printed and bound in Great Britain by MPG, Bodmin, Cornwall

Papers used by Piatkus are natural, renewable and recyclable
products made from wood grown in sustainable forests and certified
in accordance with the rules of the Forest Stewardship Council.

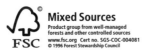

Mixed Sources
Product group from well-managed
forests and other controlled sources
www.fsc.org Cert no. SGS-COC-004081
© 1996 Forest Stewardship Council

Piatkus Books
An imprint of
Little, Brown Book Group
100 Victoria Embankment
London EC4Y 0DY

An Hachette UK Company
www.hachette.co.uk

www.piatkus.co.uk

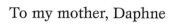
To my mother, Daphne

Contents

Acknowledgements xvii

Preface xix

Foreword xxi

Introduction 1

1. What is IVF and Do I Really Need it? 5

So, what is IVF? 6

Natural human reproduction 7

    Producing eggs 7

    Producing sperm 8

    Sexual intercourse 8

    Fertilisation 9

What can go wrong? 10

    Female fertility problems 10

    Male fertility problems 14

When can IVF help? 15

Do you need IVF? 16

Other treatments to try first 16

    Complementary therapies 18

    Keeping healthy 19

How do you feel about IVF? 19

    IVF is not for me 20

    I'm being offered IVF too soon 20

I need time to think about IVF   21
IVF is messing with nature   22
It's a means to an end   23
The stigma of IVF   23
I need to know more about IVF   24
Moving forwards   25

2. Finding the Right Clinic and Treatment for You   26

How to find the right clinic   27
    Pay a visit   27
    Success rates   28
    Waiting times   28
    Cost   29
    Treatment and eligibility   29
    Specialisms   30
    Atmosphere   30
    Location   31
    Satellite clinics   32
    Transport units   33
    Support   33
    Single women and lesbian couples 34
    Personal recommendation and reputation 35
Choosing a clinic overseas   36
Types of treatment   40
    IVF   40
    ICSI   40
    GIFT/ZIFT   41
    Natural-cycle IVF   41
    Soft, or mild, IVF   42
    IVM   42
    PGD   43
    PGS   43
    Surgical sperm retrieval – PESA, MESA, TESE 44

Assisted hatching 45
Frozen embryo transfer 46
The next step 46

3. Your First Appointment at the Clinic 47

The clinic 48
The waiting room 49
The consulting room 51
The men's room 51
The operating theatre 52
The laboratory 52
The counselling room 53
The clinic staff 53
The receptionist 53
The doctors 54
The nurses 55
The embryologists 56
Andrologists and seminologists 57
Administrative staff 58
Your first appointment 58

4. Before You Start Treatment 61

Tests 61
Rubella 62
Hepatitis B and C 62
HIV 62
Semen analysis 63
Ovarian reserve testing 63
Full blood count 64
Sexually transmitted infection tests 65
CMV-status testing 65
Ultrasound scan 65

Trial embryo transfer   65
Understanding your treatment   66
   Your drugs regime   68
   Injecting   68
Paperwork   70
Work and your impending treatment cycle   70
Telling other people   73
Ready for treatment   76

5. Preparing the Eggs   77

The drugs regime   77
   Down-regulation   78
   The stimulating drugs   79
   Scans and blood tests   80
   hCG injection   82
   Immune therapy   82
Ovarian hyperstimulation syndrome (OHSS)   84
Cancelled cycles   86
Soft, or mild, IVF   86
Egg collection   87
   The semen sample   87
   Preparing for egg collection   89
   In theatre   90

6. In the Laboratory   93

The eggs arrive in the laboratory   94
The recovery room   94
A first look at your eggs   95
   Ensuring ideal conditions in the lab   96
Preparing the sperm   96
ICSI   98
The incubators   100

Have the eggs fertilised?   101
Grading embryos   103
Blastocysts   104
Witnessing   106
Freezing and thawing   107
Preparing for embryo transfer   108

7. Embryo Transfer   109

How many embryos?   109
The embryo transfer   111
    Frozen embryo transfer   114
    Implantation and embryo transfer   115
The two-week wait   115
    Bed rest   116
    Going back to work   117
To tell or not to tell   117
    Dealing with your emotions   118
    Signs of early pregnancy   119
    Counselling and support   120
    What should and shouldn't you do during the
        two-week wait?   121

8. The Emotional Impact   125

The emotional roller coaster   125
Isolation and loneliness   126
Depression   127
Loss of control over life   128
    Putting your life on hold   129
Feelings of shame and failure   130
Personality changes   131
Relationships   132
    Dealing with other people   133

Dealing with family 134
Dealing with friends 135
When you can't have another child: emotions and
secondary infertility 136
What can you do to help yourself? 138
Communicate 138
Information 138
Support groups 140
Internet support 141
Remember the positive things in your life 143

9. Fertility Counselling 145

Types of counselling 146
Support counselling 146
Implications counselling 146
Therapeutic counselling 146
Finding a counsellor 147
What happens in a counselling session? 148
Someone to talk to 149
Privacy and counselling 150
Getting support at the start 151
Crisis points in treatment 152
Post-treatment counselling 153
Men and counselling 154
Counselling for donor gametes and surrogacy 154
Counselling is not for me 155

10. The Male Perspective 157

Male fertility problems: diagnosis 158
Treatments for male infertility 160
Vasectomy reversal 160

Using donor sperm   161
An IVF/ICSI cycle   162
  Preparing for treatment   162
  Going to the clinic   163
  IVF injections   165
Supporting your partner   166
Dealing with your own emotions   167
Dealing with other people   168
Support groups   169
Men and counselling   170

11. Using Donor Sperm and Eggs   172

Donor sperm   172
Donor eggs   174
  Egg sharing   176
Surrogacy   177
Counselling   179
  To tell or not to tell   181
IVF for single women   183
IVF for lesbian couples   185
Travelling abroad for treatment   185
Getting support   186

12. What Can You Do to Make a Difference?   188

Smoking   188
Alcohol   189
Recreational drugs   191
Weight   191
Diet   193
Supplements   194
Exercise   194

Stress   195
Lifestyle   196
Your attitude   197
Complementary therapies   198
Finding out as much as you can   198
Looking after yourself   198
The weird ones   199
Don't worry   200

13. Complementary Therapies and IVF   201

The medical point of view   202
Therapies that may help   203
   Acupuncture   203
   Traditional Chinese medicine   206
   Herbal medicine   206
   Reflexology   207
   Aromatherapy   209
   Homeopathy   210
   Hypnotherapy   211
   Craniosacral therapy   213
   Bach flower remedies   213
   Reiki   214
   Yoga   215
   Nutritional therapy   215
   Holistic fertility care   216
A note of caution   216
Men and complementary therapies   218
Cost of complementary therapies   218

14. When Treatment Doesn't Work   220

Home testing   220
Blood test   221

A low positive result 221
The negative test 222
Miscarriage 223
Ectopic pregnancy 226
Trying again after a negative result 227
Changing clinics 229
Helping yourself 230
Giving up on treatment 230

15. A Positive Pregnancy Test – Success at Last 234

The first few weeks 235
  Scans 235
  The fear of miscarriage 236
Just another pregnant woman 237
Pregnancy isn't always easy 238
Multiple pregnancy 239
Birth 239
Parenting 240

Appendix: A Brief History of IVF 242

Resources 251

International 251
Australia 252
Ireland 253
New Zealand 253
South Africa 255
United Kingdom 255
United States of America 260

Recommended Reading 261

Glossary 263
Index 267

Acknowledgements

I would like to thank everyone who took the time to speak to me for this book, especially all those who were able to be so honest about their personal experiences of IVF and infertility in order to try to help others going through the same thing. I am very grateful to the staff at fertility clinics who allowed me to spend time with them, and put up with my endless questions. I seemed to make a habit of arranging to visit on the worst possible days, so special thanks to those who were so welcoming during a power failure, and on a staff training day! My thanks to Dr Stephen Troup, Karen Schnauffer, Dawn Yell and all the staff at the Hewitt Centre at Liverpool Women's Hospital, to Helen Kendrew and everyone at the Assisted Conception Unit in Bath, to Dr Lynne Nice and Nicky Mahoney at the Chiltern Hospital and to Mike Macnamee, Dr Thomas Mathews, Rachel Holdsworth, Vivien Collins and all the staff at Bourn Hall. I had help from so many others during the long process of putting this book together, and I want to say a big thank you to Dr Luciano Nardo, Judy Boothroyd, Mollie Graneek and Sandra Hewett from the British Infertility Counselling

Association, Clare Lewis-Jones, Susan Seenan, Claire Ogilvie and all the staff and trustees of Infertility Network UK, Olivia Montuschi of the Donor Conception Network, Tony Reid and all at Fertility Friends, Karen Riley of HypnoFertility Yorkshire, Dr Lily Hua Yu of Acumedic, Susan M. Calvert – 'The Babymaker' and Elizabeth Biagi at Homeopathic Garden.

Tarek El-Toukhy generously agreed to read this book in a very early incarnation, and to act as medical adviser. He managed to wade through the chaos and offer helpful advice and suggestions for which I am most grateful. Thanks to Helen Stanton, who has been a fantastic editor and knocked the book into shape, to Denise Dwyer, to Alice Davis and Judy Piatkus for commissioning it and to my agent, Diana Tyler. Special thanks to all my friends who were horribly neglected while I wrote this, and especially to Christine Oldfield. Thank you to my mother, Daphne McCord, for all her help as ever, and to my sister, Anna McCord, whose PhD progressed in tandem with this book as we exchanged late night emails across the globe. Most of all my thanks to Max, who had so many other things to deal with but still managed to put up with me spending hours in my study, and to Alfie and Flora – yes, you really are the best children in the whole world!

Preface

Going through IVF treatment is a confusing and worrying time for many couples. Having had to deal with the difficult diagnosis of infertility, to then be presented with the need for IVF and all that entails, creates significant anxiety. There is so much to come to terms with, so many new ideas to grasp, and so many questions that need answers. Many patients often feel too afraid or embarrassed to ask, and sadly some clinicians do not always have the time to deal in detail with all the concerns that may arise. Resorting to the internet can be fraught; sifting fact from veiled advertising isn't easy.

In this book, Kate Brian presents the facts about IVF in an uncomplicated and sympathetic way. She methodically moves through each aspect of treatment, providing information on what to expect, what questions to ask and of whom, and how to deal with the rollercoaster of a treatment cycle. Besides her own experiences, which she draws upon, she includes comments and experiences of others who have been through IVF, which is likely to be helpful to readers.

Kate has been a hugely effective patient advocate in

many areas of assisted reproduction, and provides that important bridge between her specialist understanding of the technology, and being able to explain it in plain language. In this way she has provided a readable approach to a complex subject. There is a real need for this book.

Professor Peter Braude PhD FRCOG FMedSci,
Head of Department of Women's Health,
King's College London, and Consultant at
Guy's Assisted Conception Unit, London.

Foreword

Kate Brian has written a comprehensive and enlightening guide to the physical and psychological stresses imposed by IVF and related technologies. She begins by describing her own pathway through investigation and treatment, and is able to write as a consumer as well as an expert in the field. She describes her frustration at being unable to find detailed information on the experience of IVF when she was first planning to become a patient and it is to be hoped this publication will provide a useful resource to others who are coming fresh to this complicated and often challenging means of starting a family.

Throughout the book she takes care to use language which will be understood by patients as well as professionals, and explains the meaning of the many medical terms with which patients are confronted before enduring treatment. This 'IVF glossary' in itself will prove a very useful resource to patients and others interested in the process. She illustrates the various topics in the book with illustrative case histories and quotations from real patients which gives a useful practical background to the science and medicine she covers. She takes time to describe the means of choosing a clinic, perhaps one of the most important decisions that couples have to take when entering treatment, and also covers the benefits and potential problems of having treatment overseas, again well illustrated with case histories. The many and varied methods of performing IVF and related treatments are then described in detail, again providing a useful pathway for those trying to negotiate the ART minefield.

The book also describes the various members of the clinical team who work together to provide an IVF service. I think this will be new information to many patients who sometimes see the IVF doctor as the only significant person in their treatment – in fact in many ways s/he is the least important, and the book highlights the contribution made by nursing staff, embryologists and administrative staff to the overall quality of the unit. Brian then deconstructs the patient journey through IVF, from initial consultation and investigations through superovulation injections, egg collection and embryo transfer. There are many illustrative case histories which will provide prospective patients with a realistic picture of what is in store.

I was pleased to see that some of the risks associated with IVF are not understated. She takes time to describe ovarian hyperstimulation syndrome and the possible consequences for the patients, and also the risks of being asked to invest very large sums of money in treatments that are unproven. She also takes pains to discuss the risk of multiple pregnancy should multiple embryo transfer be performed and highlights the move towards single embryo transfer policy for younger patients, and the potential benefits of frozen embryo transfer.

One of the most valuable chapters is that dealing with the emotional impact of IVF treatment on couples. Brian writes with particular poignancy about this topic and uses many case histories to explore the potential harm that IVF treatment can do to relationships and psychological stability. She looks at wider issues of managing family, friends and workplace during and after treatment, and coping with the disappointment of a negative pregnancy test after IVF treatment. A number of strategies are suggested to help future patients cope with these pressures, and support systems are identified.

The central place of counselling in good quality IVF treatment is emphasised and the importance of seeing a counsellor who has specific interest and knowledge in the area is highlighted. She points out some of the crisis points in treatment, and also the need to consider the male partner in the counselling process. Indeed, the role of the male is dealt with in detail – an often neglected topic but one which will be of considerable importance to the couples reading the book before treatment. Those men who find the prospect of reading through the whole book daunting should be directed specifically to this chapter, as it contains much wisdom.

One of the controversial areas in IVF treatment is the use of donor gametes or embryos, particularly since this often involves travel overseas due to the mismatch between demand and supply for donated gametes in the United Kingdom. Brian deals with some of the risks involved with overseas travel for gamete donation, again handling the topic with balance and sensitivity and giving useful information for those contemplating the process. She goes on to describe methods of 'self help' to try and improve chances of pregnancy from IVF treatment, including a critical look at the field of complementary therapy and IVF, and a caveat concerning the high cost of some treatment in some centres. Complementary therapy is dealt with in depth, with description of the whole range of therapies available and their potential benefits.

Brian concludes with a chapter that describes the process following a pregnancy test – whether positive or negative, and how to cope with a negative test after considerable investment of time, energy and sometimes finance. She is careful to highlight the risks of ectopic pregnancy and miscarriage which can still surprise patients after IVF treatment has resulted in a positive pregnancy test.

I enjoyed reading this book. As a professional involved with IVF treatment in daily working life I found it useful to see ART from the patients' perspective. I would certainly recommend the book to anyone struggling with infertility or considering IVF treatment and I can envisage patients turning back to it at the various stages of their treatment pathway as a useful source of reference.

Professor William Ledger, Academic Unit of Reproductive and Developmental Medicine, University of Sheffield

Introduction

No one wants to have IVF, but if you're reading this book the chances are that either you, or someone close to you, is finding it hard to get pregnant naturally and may be facing the prospect of fertility treatment. We like to imagine that IVF is something that happens to other people, and hope that we'll be pregnant long before we get that far down the line, but since IVF started in the 1970s thousands of people around the world have found that it can offer the hope of a solution to their fertility problems.

This book aims to give you a clear idea of what is involved in IVF treatment. You may understand the medical procedures, you may have spent a lot of time finding out about other people's experiences, but you probably don't know so much about what goes on behind the scenes during an IVF cycle, about the people involved in treatment and about their perspective on the process. The more insight you have into IVF, the less daunting it will seem.

I'm only too aware of how alarming the prospect of going through IVF can be. I was 30 when we started trying to have a baby. We had always known we wanted a family one day, but once we finally felt the time was right and began looking forward to having children of our own, we found we couldn't conceive. Month after month passed, and I decided to take the matter in hand, expecting to be able to find a cause and a solution for the problem fairly rapidly. Instead, I soon learned there are rarely easy answers or quick fixes when it comes to infertility.

Our infertility remained unexplained despite endless tests, and eventually it was suggested that IVF might be the best way ahead. I was still hoping I would miraculously get pregnant naturally at the last minute, but in the meantime I set about finding out all I could about what would be involved. At the time the Internet was still in its infancy, and there wasn't the easy access we have now to research, information, and, perhaps more importantly, to the experiences of other people who have already been through fertility treatment themselves.

I read everything I could find, but it was virtually impossible to discover what IVF would be like for me as a patient, and that's how I ended up writing my first book on the subject, *In Pursuit of Parenthood*, about patients' experiences of assisted conception. I'd already had my first unsuccessful attempt at IVF followed by an unsuccessful frozen embryo transfer when I wrote the proposal for the book, and by the time it was commissioned I was pregnant after another fresh IVF cycle.

I learned more about the issues involved as I met fertility experts, and spoke to other patients, and I became a trustee of the charity, CHILD, which has since merged with another patient group to become

Infertility Network UK. Although I had a baby, I was still very aware that I was unable to conceive naturally. I had secretly hoped we would be one of those couples with unexplained infertility who go on to have children naturally following successful IVF, but after a couple of years we had to accept it wasn't going to happen, and went back to the fertility clinic.

We still had embryos in the freezer, and we worked our way through them, and had another unsuccessful fresh IVF treatment before our fifth frozen embryo cycle led to a positive pregnancy test, and the birth of our daughter. By this time, I had given up my job in television news and became more involved in the fertility field. I'd worked on a number of projects with Infertility Network UK, and had written articles about infertility for newspapers and magazines. I was frequently asked to give a patient's perspective on fertility stories in the news for journalists and broadcasters, and at conferences for doctors and nurses as well as patients. I was also invited to join an expert advisory group at the Human Fertilisation and Embryology Authority looking into multiple births after fertility treatment.

I was becoming increasingly aware that one of the burning issues for women today was how late they could risk leaving it to have a baby. This was why I came to write my last book, *The Complete Guide to Female Fertility*, which covers the medical, social and emotional aspects of the subject, and addresses the thorny issue of the biological clock.

While writing *The Complete Guide to Female Fertility* I realised that although it is far easier to find out about IVF nowadays, there is still a lot of mystique associated with the process, and there is often a wide gulf between the patients who have the treatment and the staff working in the clinics who treat them. Patients often have no idea what goes on behind the scenes, and don't always feel confident about asking questions or raising issues that concern them. This book is an attempt to make the process less alien and to try to give an honest and understandable view of what happens during an IVF cycle from all perspectives.

I hope this book will help you feel more confident about fertility treatment as it guides you through the process. No one can fully appreciate what it is like to experience infertility and IVF unless they have been there themselves, but you will discover that most of us who have trodden the path are only too willing to do anything we can to help you along the way, and to share our experiences in the hope that it might make it a little easier for you.

Chapter one

What is IVF and Do I Really Need it?

We grow up believing that we will be able to have a family when we decide the time is right, and most of our education about fertility focuses on ensuring we know how to prevent unplanned pregnancies. It can come as a surprise to learn how common it is for couples to have problems conceiving, and how many things can go wrong.

Although we may have heard of IVF, we don't expect it to come into our lives. Even when we find ourselves failing to conceive month after month after month, we still assume that IVF would be a last resort, and hope that we will be offered some other, less complicated, solution. The reality is that more and more of us are having to consider IVF if we want to have children of our own, and it's not until we reach that point that we discover quite how little we know about what is involved.

So, what is IVF?

IVF is a form of assisted conception used to help people with fertility problems. The initials stand for *in vitro* fertilisation, and during IVF eggs are fertilised in the laboratory, rather than inside the female body as would happen naturally. The term *in vitro* means 'in glass', and so people often assume embryos are created in glass test-tubes during IVF, which led to the expression 'test-tube babies'. In fact, eggs, sperm and embryos are kept in plastic dishes in the laboratory, and the phrase *in vitro* has a more general meaning of 'in an artificial situation', or outside the body.

In simple terms, IVF involves taking eggs from a woman's ovaries, and mixing them with sperm in a dish. If a sperm breaks into the egg and fertilises it, it will become an embryo. If all goes well, one or more embryos can be transferred to the womb, where it is hoped they will flourish and result in a pregnancy.

Each attempt at IVF is called a cycle, and drugs are usually prescribed as part of the treatment to allow the doctors to take control of the woman's hormones in order to produce more than one egg. Most women will produce only one mature egg at a time in their natural menstrual cycle, but the drugs used in IVF stimulate the ovaries so that they churn out a number of eggs to maximise the chances that some will be fertilised and result in a pregnancy.

Natural human reproduction

It is probably helpful to start by considering how both male and female bodies should work, as this will help us to understand where things can go wrong in natural reproduction, and why IVF might be necessary.

A fertile woman releases an egg from one of her ovaries each month, and a fertile male is constantly making more sperm. If the couple have intercourse around the time an egg is released, sperm can travel from the vagina up through the neck of the womb – called the cervix – and fertilise the egg.

Producing eggs

A woman must be making eggs and then releasing them (or ovulating) if an egg is to be fertilised this way. Women usually start ovulating when they reach puberty and will carry on having periods until they reach the menopause, although their fertility will decline many years before this.

Egg production is regulated by hormones, and in order for the eggs to start to grow inside their little fluid-filled sacs (called follicles) in the ovary, a woman has to produce follicle-stimulating hormone, known as FSH. At the same time, the lining of the womb, or endometrium, starts to grow thicker and spongy, preparing it for a fertilised egg to nestle down, or implant, and continue to grow.

Once the FSH has stimulated the follicles, more and more of another hormone, oestrogen, is produced. When the oestrogen reaches a certain level, it is time for the egg to be released. It normally takes about 14 days to reach this point in the cycle, but it varies from woman to woman. As soon as the egg is ready, the body produces a huge surge of luteinising hormone, or LH, and that triggers ovulation, when the egg bursts out of the follicle. Once the egg is released, it begins the journey towards the womb, travelling down a thin tube, the fallopian tube, that connects each ovary to the womb.

Producing sperm

Men make millions of sperm every single day, starting when they reach puberty. Although the process slows down as they get older, most men will still be able to produce viable sperm that can fertilise an egg when they are collecting their pensions.

Like the female egg-releasing cycle, sperm production is controlled by the hormones. People often imagine that testosterone, the hormone responsible for sex drive, must also be responsible for sperm production, but most of the work is done by the same two hormones that control much of the female cycle: FSH and LH. Unlike women, men produce both these hormones all the time, and it is the FSH that stimulates the production of sperm in the testicles. Sperm production takes more than 60 days, as the sperm have to mature and grow in order to be capable of breaking into an egg and fertilising it. Mature sperm are stored in the testicles and at the upper end of the tubes that lead down into the penis.

Sexual intercourse

During intercourse, semen is ejaculated into the vagina. Just a tiny percentage of the semen is made up of sperm. The rest is seminal fluid that carries the sperm safely from the testicles to the vagina. Although only one sperm is needed to fertilise an egg, there will be millions in the ejaculate. Most of them are killed almost instantly by the acid conditions of the vagina, but a few hundred may make it to the cervix. If this happens around the time the woman is ovulating, the mucus around her cervix will have become watery and thin, making it easy for the sperm to swim up into the womb. Once inside the female body, sperm can live for up to a week, although most won't last longer than a couple of days.

Fertilisation

Once the surviving sperm reach the womb they keep swimming upwards and head towards the fallopian tubes. If an egg has recently been released from the ovary, it will be travelling down the tubes towards them. The sperm will normally fertilise the egg in the tube rather than in the womb.

The sperm will head for both the tubes, but as only one egg is produced at a time, many of them will have swum off in the wrong direction towards an empty tube. It's quite hard for them to keep travelling upwards once they get into the tube, as it is lined with tiny hair-like cilia, that are waving the egg down towards the womb in the opposite direction.

The outer coating surrounding the sperm's head is stripped off as it passes through the tube (in a process known as capacitation), which will help the sperm to fertilise the egg, and the tail starts making very wide beats. Dozens of sperm are travelling up the tube at the same time, and each will try to be first to break through the outer coating and bind itself to the egg. As soon as one sperm manages this, enzymes immediately act on the shell of the egg to make it into a hard barrier so that no others can get in. If more than one sperm does enter an egg, the egg will not survive.

The fertilised egg begins dividing a day later, first into two cells, then into four cells and again to make eight. Soon the fertilised egg, or embryo, will be ready to implant itself into the soft lining of the womb and grow.

What can go wrong?

As we've seen, natural human reproduction is a complex process, and there are many stages during which things can go wrong. A small upset at any point along the way can prevent conception, and when a couple are experiencing fertility problems, it can take time for doctors to work out exactly where the difficulty may lie.

Female fertility problems

Women may have to go through a barrage of tests in order to get to the root of a female fertility problem, which may be hormonal or physical.

Hormonal problems are often to blame, as an imbalance in the hormones that regulate egg production and ovulation can mean that eggs are not produced every month, or that they are not released at all, or that they do not develop properly.

Polycystic ovary syndrome (often known as PCOS) is a common cause of female fertility problems, as it can disrupt ovulation. Although more than 20 per cent of women have polycystic ovaries, where there are undeveloped follicles (or cysts) just under the surface of the ovaries, these are often not accompanied by any other symptoms and don't affect fertility. In women who have polycystic ovary syndrome, however, there are a number of other symptoms. The menstrual cycle is often affected and ovulation is usually irregular, infrequent or entirely absent.

About a third of women with PCOS are overweight, and they may also have unwanted facial or body hair, and skin problems such as oily skin or acne. The hormonal imbalances often associated with PCOS mean women may produce higher than normal levels of testosterone and insulin, the hormone that regulates blood sugar levels. PCOS can affect women who have eating disorders, and if you have bulimia you are at risk of developing PCOS even if your weight is normal.

An early or premature menopause, which happens when the ovaries stop functioning properly many years before they should, occurs in about 2 per cent of women. It can take place when women are still in their twenties, and the causes are not always clear, although they may be genetic or chromosomal. Women who've had an early menopause will usually be able to get pregnant only by using donated eggs, as once a woman reaches the menopause, the process is irreversible.

Raised prolactin levels can disrupt ovulation, and women who have high prolactin levels may have irregular periods, or none at all. Prolactin is a hormone that helps prepare women's breasts for milk production after childbirth, but levels can sometimes rise in women who are not pregnant and this can affect their hormonal balance.

Endometriosis, a condition where tissue similar to the womb lining starts growing elsewhere around the reproductive organs, can cause female fertility problems. It is very common, affecting around 15 per cent of women. Many women who have endometriosis still get pregnant without any difficulty, but others will find it affects their ability to conceive. It may be accompanied by heavy, painful periods and pain in the abdomen, lower back or pelvis.

Fibroids are benign tumours made up of muscle fibre that grow in or around the womb. They may make it difficult for a fertilised embryo to implant successfully and they are also associated with miscarriage. Many women who have fibroids are completely unaware of them, but they may be accompanied by heavy menstrual bleeding, painful periods, bloating or lower back pain.

Problems with the fallopian tubes are another common cause of infertility. The fallopian tubes lead from the ovaries to the womb, and if they are blocked, scarred or damaged, this may stop an egg travelling along them. The tubes can be damaged by infection, or by scar tissue if you've had surgery in the pelvic area. One major cause of tubal problems nowadays is the sexually transmitted infection, chlamydia. It can lead to pelvic inflammatory disease, which damages the fallopian tubes. Chlamydia is extremely common and it is estimated that around 10 per cent of sexually active young people have the infection, which is passed on through unprotected intercourse.

There are often no outward signs, so a woman may be completely unaware that she has chlamydia although it may be putting her future fertility at risk.

A hydrosalpinx is the medical term for a fluid-filled blockage in the fallopian tubes. This can happen when one of the tubes gets completely blocked as a result of infection or scarring, and fills up with fluid. Some women who have a hydrosalpinx find it extremely painful, whereas others have no symptoms at all. In some cases, both tubes get blocked at the same time and this is referred to as bilateral hydrosalpinges. If you have a hydrosalpinx, doctors often advise removing the tube entirely before having IVF, as it is thought to affect the chances of an embryo implanting and increase the risk of miscarriage.

Physical problems with the womb or ovaries can make it difficult to conceive. Sometimes the outer surface of the ovaries may be scarred and this can affect ovulation. The womb can be unusually shaped, or scarred, which may lead to fertility problems.

Age is a crucial factor in female fertility, as the biological clock limits our ability to conceive. Women start to become less fertile when they are in their thirties, and female fertility declines sharply once a woman reaches her forties. Although some women continue to have periods until they reach their early fifties, their fertility is compromised for some years before their periods stop and they reach the menopause. Age-related fertility problems are common today, as more women are starting their families later in life.

People often assume that fertility treatment will overcome age-related fertility problems, but the chances of success using assisted conception are directly related to your age in just the same way that they are with natural conception. Although IVF success rates have risen over the years, the rates for women over 40 have remained low.

Secondary infertility occurs when women who have already had one child, or even two children, without any problems encounter them when trying to get pregnant again. Things can change in your body with time, and with age, and a fertility problem that you were able to overcome in your early thirties may not be so easy to conquer when combined with your decreasing fertility in your early forties. Couples sometimes delay seeking medical help if they've already had a child, assuming that nothing could be wrong, but having had one child is not a guarantee that you will be able to have another.

Unexplained infertility is surprisingly common, and many couples will never discover why they're having problems conceiving. All the tests may come back suggesting there is absolutely nothing wrong, and although some unexplained infertility could be linked to age, in most cases it is just that no cause has been found with the tests we now have available.

Male fertility problems

Most male factor fertility problems are to do with sperm production. When a man gives a semen sample for analysis, there should be at least twenty million sperm per millilitre of semen. If there are fewer than this, a man may be told that he has a low sperm count, or fewer sperm than normal in his semen.

It isn't just the quantity of sperm that is important but also the quality. The sperm need to be able to swim forwards fairly quickly if they are to fertilise an egg. If the sperm are very sluggish, or if they swim in circles, this is referred to as a motility problem and it may hamper fertilisation. Sometimes the sperm haven't formed properly, or are abnormally shaped, and they are then said to have poor morphology. Most semen samples contain some abnormal sperm, and it is only if too many are misshapen or unable to swim normally that it causes real problems.

Some men have no sperm in the semen at all. This might mean that none are being produced in the testicles, but it often occurs when there is a blockage in the tube leading down to the penis or if the tube hasn't developed properly.

When can IVF help?

Originally, IVF was developed to help women who had blocked or damaged fallopian tubes to get pregnant. As it involves taking eggs directly from the ovaries, and putting embryos back into the womb, it bypasses the tubes completely, and has always been particularly good for helping women with tubal problems.

Nowadays, IVF is far more widely used for a variety of female fertility problems, including difficulties with ovulation, endometriosis and unexplained infertility. As the IVF process has developed, it can now be used more often for male fertility problems, too.

Do you need IVF?

Sometimes, couples know fairly soon after they start having fertility tests that they will need IVF if they are ever going to have a child, and the situation is clear cut. For others, however, it is not so straightforward, particularly where no cause has been found for the fertility problems.

When you're going through the initial phase of tests, things can drag terribly, with weeks or even months between appointments, and you may feel that you are spending most of your time waiting. However, once you get into the next stage, it can seem as if you are catapulted into IVF, without having had time to think properly about whether it is something you really want or need.

Other treatments to try first

Not everyone has concerns about IVF, but if you do, you may want to reassure yourself that you are sure you have tried every alternative option first. There are some other treatments you may be offered before IVF, but they may not always be appropriate for everyone. The type of treatment suggested will depend on the nature of the fertility problem.

Drug treatments may be offered for hormonal problems, as these can help regulate the female menstrual cycle and ovulation. Drugs are sometimes, although far less often, prescribed where there is a male-factor problem to try to improve the sperm count.

Laparoscopic ovarian drilling may sometimes be suggested for women with polycystic ovaries. This involves an operation during which small holes are made in the surface of the ovaries. This process seems to help trigger ovulation in some women.

Surgery can be an option for women with tubal problems, although IVF tends to be seen as a more successful way of achieving a pregnancy in such cases. Surgery may also be used to remove fibroids or scar tissue from the womb, and may help with some male-factor problems.

If a man or woman has been sterilised in the past to prevent pregnancy, surgeons can try to reverse the operation. However, attempting to re-join the female fallopian tubes, or to mend the tubes that carry sperm from the testicles to the penis once they've been cut or blocked is a delicate surgical process and it is not always successful.

Intrauterine insemination, or IUI, may be attempted before launching into IVF, as it is a cheaper and less invasive treatment. IUI is a form of artificial insemination, where sperm are inserted into the womb around the time of ovulation, and fertilisation takes place inside the woman's body.

Sometimes, IUI is carried out in a natural cycle, which means the female partner doesn't take any drugs at all. She will be monitored to check when she is about to release an egg, and may use an ovulation prediction kit to pinpoint the right moment for the sperm to be transferred. If there are any problems with ovulation, or if a number of natural cycle treatments haven't worked, the medical team may suggest using drugs to stimulate the ovaries, and this is known as a stimulated cycle. Close monitoring is essential in stimulated cycles, to make sure that the ovaries don't produce too many eggs, which could lead to a multiple pregnancy.

The male partner produces a semen sample by masturbation, and the best-quality sperm are filtered out. They are put into a thin tube, which is inserted into the vagina and passed through the neck of the womb. The sperm are then injected into the womb itself.

IUI tends to be much less successful than IVF, as it is a fairly simple treatment, and some couples, therefore, feel it is a waste of time and want to move straight on to IVF. IVF is more expensive and invasive, but it does allow doctors to see how the eggs and sperm work together, as they can monitor fertilisation in the laboratory. Not everyone wants to rush into IVF, and some people feel they would prefer to give everything else a good chance first. Your decision may be influenced by the nature of the fertility problem, and your age and financial situation, and you should discuss it with your doctor or nurse if you have any uncertainties about when would be the right time for you to move on to IVF.

Complementary therapies

It is increasingly common for couples with fertility problems to use complementary therapies, and some practitioners make bold claims about their methods and success rates. There are undoubtedly many people who feel that complementary therapies have played an important role in helping them to conceive, and these treatments may help you feel more relaxed and reduce your stress levels. Complementary therapies may be helpful for infertility when they are used alongside conventional medicine in a truly complementary, rather than alternative, manner, and if you are interested in this I have included a chapter on their use later in the book.

Keeping healthy

Some couples find that making lifestyle changes will improve their chances of getting pregnant naturally. If you are very overweight, if you smoke or drink a lot of alcohol, then looking at how you can make changes here first will help you ensure they're not causing problems.

Anyone trying to conceive should also be taking folic acid, as this can help prevent serious birth defects if you get pregnant. When you've been trying to conceive for month after month, or year after year, you may feel it is pointless to keep on taking folic acid, but it is particularly important in the first few weeks of pregnancy so it is vital to continue taking it, even if you think it is unlikely that you are going to conceive naturally.

How do you feel about IVF?

IVF is something most of us imagine is for other people. We expect that we'll somehow manage to conceive before we get that far down the line of fertility treatment, and you may find you feel quite alarmed when IVF is first mentioned as an option.

IVF is not for me

Some couples start out on their fertility journey feeling absolutely adamant that IVF is not for them. It may be that after trying other treatments without success, you don't want to go any further down the route of assisted conception. Fertility treatment is tough, and it can become overwhelming. There are people who would prefer to face a life without children, or perhaps consider adoption, rather than allowing their entire lives to be dominated by their fertility problems. This is a perfectly valid decision to make, but you may face pressure from friends or family who have no idea what it is like to go through treatment and who may feel you should persevere. Remember that this is your decision, and only you know how you will feel about it.

Although some people remain certain that they won't ever get embroiled in IVF, others may find they have a change of heart once they realise it could be the only way they will ever have a child of their own. What can seem a horrendous prospect from the safe distance of assuming that you are going to get pregnant naturally may suddenly become far more acceptable if it becomes a choice between IVF and childlessness. No one expects to have IVF, but as you learn more about it, you realise quite how widely it is used to help with fertility problems. Already, more than three and a half million people have been conceived this way worldwide.

I'm being offered IVF too soon

Even those who don't have any particular problem with IVF can feel it has arrived as an option sooner than they had anticipated, because most of us hope we will get pregnant before we need IVF. I'd always envisaged IVF as something you would contemplate only in dire circumstances if everything else had failed, and although we'd been through years of tests and fertility drugs, I hadn't realised we were getting close to that stage.

Some doctors do feel that IVF is often offered to couples too quickly, and this is partly because other methods may be time-consuming and less successful. Toni and her partner had unexplained infertility, and they expected to spend some time trying other treatments before launching into IVF. In fact, their clinic suggested it fairly early on, as Toni explains:

> I was a bit surprised that they suggested going for IVF. When I first went to the clinic, they said they'd try about four rounds of IUI first, but I hadn't heard of a lot of success from it so I was happy to go with IVF, although I thought I was a long way off doing it. I was worried that it was going to be mentally and physically challenging.

Patients can feel shocked and surprised when the prospect of IVF is first mooted. Helena's doctors had found no reason why she couldn't get pregnant, and she hadn't anticipated being offered IVF for some time: 'I went in for a review, and they said they thought the quickest way for me to get pregnant was probably IVF. I always knew it was an option, but nobody had ever said it was necessarily likely. I felt absolutely stunned.'

I need time to think about IVF
It may take you a while to feel happy about going forward with IVF, and it is important to give yourself the time

to think it through. You are going to be making a big emotional, and probably financial, commitment, and you need to feel ready. Sometimes people find they are suddenly worried about things they hadn't even thought of before, and if this happens to you, you may want to address these concerns and talk them through with the medical team or counsellor.

I'm not sure anyone ever feels completely prepared for IVF, but some people do find it easier to make the decision to go ahead than others. Lulu admits it took her a long time to come to terms with the idea:

I was very worried because I was quite into alternative things, and I'd always wanted to try and get pregnant without going to such drastic lengths. It seemed like the last port of call. I was worried about side effects of the drugs, and I was worried about failure – what if you go through all that, spend all that money, and it doesn't work?

IVF is messing with nature

We still have this image of IVF as a rather mysterious high-tech treatment, and so much of the media coverage has been warped by visions of human cloning, hybrid embryos and designer babies that we sometimes have quite muddled ideas of what will be involved. People may have religious objections to assisted reproduction; for example, the Roman Catholic Church is opposed to IVF, and some Muslims would not want to use donor eggs or sperm.

I was filled with doubts when we were about to start our first IVF cycle. Taking eggs from my body and fertilising them in a laboratory seemed such an unnatural way of creating life, and I found myself wondering whether I should accept our infertility as fate, rather than trying to interfere with nature. A lot of the criticisms of fertility treatment focus on this idea of doctors 'playing God', but it is important to remember that during IVF you are simply creating the right circumstances for fertilisation. The real miracles of why some eggs fertilise, implant in the womb and grow are still all down to nature.

It's a means to an end

Some people find they are surprisingly calm and relaxed about IVF. It's great if you can see it simply as a step towards what you want, but it may be hard to maintain that sense of calm rationality throughout the ups and downs of a treatment cycle. Kate was waiting for her first treatment cycle when we spoke, and had managed to detach herself emotionally, but admitted she wasn't sure she would be able to maintain that as she got further down the line: 'I see it as a means to an end. I am very practical about it. If it works, it works and if it doesn't, I have tried. I am quite chilled about the whole thing, but I don't suppose I will be when it comes to starting the treatment.'

The stigma of IVF

There can be a sense of shame associated with infertility, and you may find you feel some stigma about the fact that you need help to have a child. The fact that infertility and IVF are so common doesn't make it any easier for an individual to deal with these emotions, or to get over them.

Sometimes there has been an element of denial about

our infertility during the months or years of tests and treatment leading up to this point, and it is only when we find ourselves face to face with IVF that we have to accept that we are not going to conceive in the normal way. This may be the first time we have had to acknowledge the reality of our fertility problems, and it is not always easy. I had hoped that we would somehow manage to conceive before we started IVF, and right up to the moment I began taking the drugs I was still hoping that I would be one of the people you read about who get pregnant at the last minute once they have signed up for treatment. It can happen and it does happen, but once you've got to this stage, it is far more likely that it won't.

I need to know more about IVF

When you're told you should consider IVF, you may suddenly realise how little you know about it. There are some people who like it this way; those who prefer not to know any more than they absolutely need to, and who are happy to plunge in, feeling that the more they know, the more they will worry. However, many people do find that reading and researching gives an understanding of what is going to happen, and makes them feel more in control. This is a matter of personal choice, and sometimes one partner wants to know all they can whereas the other may cope by trying to ignore what is happening.

Joining a support network or an Internet forum can be helpful, as you will be able to find out about other people's experiences of treatment. Occasionally, people do report that reading too much of other people's experiences has made them worry unnecessarily and expect the worst, so you may want to bear this in mind, because you may not find IVF as tough as some other people do.

Moving forwards

Once you've accepted that you are going to try IVF as a possible route to parenthood, you may feel far more positive. After years of trying to get pregnant unsuccessfully, there may be relief and excitement that at last you are finally doing something about it, that your situation is being taken seriously, and that you are going to put yourself in the hands of a team of experts who will be working with you to try to reach your goal.

What can be particularly difficult once you've decided to try IVF, is dealing with your expectations. When you're investing so much time, effort, and usually money too, into your treatment, you may feel that it ought to work. It is worth remembering that most people who have had their families through IVF didn't get pregnant the first time they tried it. When you look at the figures for those who've continued with treatment, the chances of success improve considerably.

I hope that this book will give you the knowledge that will help you feel less worried and nervous about IVF. It is never going to be an easy thing to go through, but I believe that if you know what to expect, and if you are aware of what is going on at each stage of your treatment, it will help you feel more in control, and the process will seem less daunting.

Chapter two

Finding the Right Clinic and Treatment for You

If you know you're going to need assisted conception, you will want to be sure you are having the right kind of treatment and at the right place for you. For some people, these decisions are straightforward; you may know that IVF is what you need, and have just one clinic nearby that offers it. For others, there may be a wide choice of clinics, or you may not be sure whether IVF alone will be able to do the trick. Whatever the case, you will want to be as informed as you can before making any decisions.

When we started on the IVF route, we had a wide range of clinics to choose from, but having spent some time researching their relative merits, we ended up basing our choice on the fact that one particular consultant came highly recommended by a work colleague. His clinic was new, and success rates were not established, but we liked and trusted the staff, it was an easy journey from our home, there was no waiting list and the treatment was affordable. Only you can tell which are the things that are going to matter to you, but you will want to be sure you're looking at the right details, whether you're phoning around clinics, going to visit, or checking them out online.

How to find the right clinic

When you're trying to find a clinic, trawling the Internet can leave you with pages of information about the types of treatment on offer, success rates, clinic staff and prices. It can all seem rather overwhelming, so I've listed some key factors you may want to take into consideration when making your decision.

Pay a visit

If you have a choice, it's always a good idea to visit a few clinics first. Many clinics now have open days, or special sessions for patients who are thinking of having treatment, and one consultant I spoke to said it was always advisable to have a look before you make a decision:

> We encourage patients to look at a range of clinics and to choose the one that is most appropriate to them. We offer a free informal visit where the prospective patients can come in and have a chat. It's not about anything clinical, but about important things like our opening times and how many times they'll need to come in, so that they can see whether it will fit in with their work patterns.

Success rates

The key factor in most people's decision-making process when it comes to choosing a clinic is its success rate. Generally, this is a reasonable way to make an assessment of how well the clinic does, but you should be aware that the overall clinic success rate is not necessarily the same as your individual chance of having a baby at that particular clinic. The chances of success depend on the age of the patient, and the duration and nature of the fertility problem. Also, success rates may vary from one year to another.

Success rates are affected by the clientele of the clinic, and if lots of the patients are arriving after repeated unsuccessful attempts elsewhere, this will make a difference to the outcomes. The general health of the patients might make a difference, too, and an expensive private clinic treating otherwise healthy patients at the top of the socio-economic scale is likely to do better than a clinic in a deprived area. In some cases, a clinic with a slightly lower overall success rate may offer a better chance of success at your age and with your fertility problem.

Waiting times

The time you'll have to wait to get an appointment at the clinic, and the length of the waiting list for treatment, may play a role in your choice of clinics. If you are hoping to have funded treatment, rather than paying to go privately, this may mean an even longer waiting list. This may be particularly important to you if you are very aware that your age is working against you, and know that treatment is likely to be less successful the longer you have to wait. There are often long waiting times for those who need to use donor eggs or sperm.

Cost

You may be fortunate and have some of your treatment funded, but the cost of treatment is a major issue for many people. Fertility treatment is not cheap, and some clinics charge more than others. Not all give a clearly costed estimate at the start of how much you should expect to pay in total. It is essential to make sure you have looked into this before you start, as there can be unexpected extras if you haven't clarified things with the clinic. Check whether there could be any additional tests that haven't been included, and whether the total takes into account the cost of drugs. If you find there are going to be any extras, make sure you get estimates for these, too. You should also find out what the cost is for freezing and storing any spare embryos, as this can be another expense you may not have factored into your budget.

Treatment and eligibility

Some fertility clinics offer only a limited range of fertility treatments, and you may want to check what the clinic can provide before you start. There are sometimes restrictions on eligibility for treatment that can vary considerably from clinic to clinic. Most will set upper age limits, and many refuse to treat women who are very overweight. Not all clinics have the right facilities to treat patients who test positive for HIV or hepatitis, and this may limit your choices considerably. If you suspect any of these could be an issue, it is worth checking before you get to the stage of paying for an initial consultation.

Kate realised herself that she was going to have to lose weight if she wanted to have IVF:

It was only mentioned once, and the consultant didn't say you need to lose weight, she just said if you're going to do IVF, your Body Mass Index has to be under 35. Mine was 41. By the time the referral had come through I had lost nearly six stone, so my weight was nearly what it needed to be.

Specialisms

If you know you have a specific problem, you may want to find out whether there are any consultants in your area who specialise in that field. Medical teams at fertility clinics will have the knowledge and expertise to deal with every type of problem, but some doctors concentrate their research on particular aspects of infertility, and may be more skilled, and successful, at helping those with certain conditions.

Atmosphere

Over the years, I've visited dozens of fertility clinics and I've come to realise quite how different in terms of atmosphere they can be. I've been to grand clinics with chandeliers and staircases curving upwards from vast tiled hallways, shabby clinics in tired hospitals that have seen better days, tiny clinics jammed into rooms scarcely bigger than oversized cupboards, and huge, busy clinics with large waiting rooms packed with patients. Each of us will have our own individual reactions to the atmosphere of a clinic, and what suits one person may not be right for another, although the treatment will be broadly the same wherever you go.

Some people prefer the businesslike impersonality of many of the larger clinics, where success rates are often high and the treatment process is carried out with brisk efficiency. Others find this off-putting, and may prefer the more relaxed atmosphere of a smaller clinic where you will get to know the staff, and they will get to know you. Some would baulk at a unit situated in a sprawling run-down hospital, whereas others have reported feeling overawed by the elegant luxury of some private clinics. You will know what suits you best, and although atmosphere may sound an absurd basis for making a choice of clinic, it isn't a factor you should instantly dismiss. If you feel comfortable where you are being treated, it is going to make the treatment process far easier to deal with, and that can make all the difference.

Lulu had to choose between two local clinics – one very large and successful, and the other much smaller:

> The large clinic has a fantastic reputation and great success rates, but it felt like it was a bit of a factory. There were so many people going though the system, and it felt impersonal. Then I went to the smaller clinic and something said to me when I walked in that it was the right place. It had a very good feeling, and I felt comfortable. I knew if I felt comfortable I would be more relaxed, which could only help the whole process.

Location

The choices you have when it comes to fertility clinics may depend on your geographical location. Large cities are often home to a number of units, but in remote rural areas, there may be only one option within a reasonable travelling distance.

You will need to visit the clinic on a fairly regular basis during your treatment, and you should take the journey into consideration. What seems feasible for an occasional visit may become exhausting when you have to do the journey three times in one week, and it can make your experience of treatment much easier if you have a short and straightforward trip.

If you feel your local clinic doesn't have acceptable success rates, or if it doesn't offer the treatment options you need, or simply doesn't feel right for you, it would be foolish to compromise your chances of success and the way you are going to feel about the experience purely on the basis of location, but you do need to be realistic about how you will manage if you have a very long journey.

Sandra and her husband went to their local clinic for most of their treatment, but changed for their most recent cycle to another clinic much further from home:

It's a four-hour trip by the time I get to our new clinic and back, and I had to go twice a week and take the whole day off work. The original clinic we went to was good, but we chose it because it was five minutes from where we live. I do feel confident we've chosen the right place this time, whereas before I think we chose the location over everything else and we shouldn't have done.

Satellite clinics

Some larger fertility centres have links with other smaller units, or with gynaecology departments in local hospitals, and will work together during IVF treatment. If you attend a satellite unit, they will carry out the monitoring part of the cycle, and then you will transfer to the main fertility clinic for egg collection and embryo transfer.

Isobel lives in an area with no local fertility centre. She had treatment at a satellite unit close to her home, and then had to fly to the nearest hospital offering IVF. Isobel explains: 'The consultant at the local hospital prescribes the drugs that the clinic set, and she does all the scans. You just go away for the egg collection and embryo transfer.'

Transport units

A transport unit works on the same principle as a satellite clinic, but they actually carry out the egg collection locally as well. Once the eggs have been collected, they have to be taken to the embryology lab at the main fertility clinic. It is usually up to the woman's partner to do that, as the head of one IVF clinic that works with transport units explains:

> We have shared care with the transport units. The eggs have to be in the custody of the patient, so the bloke comes in with the eggs and sperm. They carry them in an incubator about the size of a large vanity case, which you plug into the cigarette lighter in the car. The couple come to the clinic for embryo transfer, and then we pass care back to their clinic.

It all sounds quite extraordinary – transporting the eggs and sperm in a case plugged into your cigarette lighter – but as long as the eggs are kept safely in their incubator at the correct temperature, being moved this way doesn't do them any harm.

Support

All fertility clinics should offer counselling, but some do it with far more enthusiasm than others. There may be a resident counsellor who has his, or her, own room at the clinic, or you may have to visit a counsellor affiliated to the clinic who works from consulting rooms at another location. If the clinic is less supportive, you may simply be given a phone number to call if you need counselling, and be expected to arrange it yourself.

You may want to check whether there is a patient support group at the clinic. As more and more patients contact one another online, clinics often feel there isn't the demand for support groups. In fact, there's a lot to be said for meeting one another face to face, and this kind of support can be particularly helpful.

Single women and lesbian couples

Even relatively recently, some clinics were less than enthusiastic about offering IVF to lesbian couples or single women, but attitudes have changed considerably and it is now generally understood that there are discrimination issues involved here. There are clinics that have always had a more liberal standpoint on this issue, and although this won't affect the outcome of your treatment, it is possible that it may affect your experience as a patient having IVF at the clinic. If you are a single woman, or a lesbian couple, and you feel this could be an issue, it is a good idea to have a chat with someone at the clinic before you begin, to gauge how frequently they treat single women and lesbians, and how they feel about it.

Annabel had a hard time finding a clinic that would treat her as a single woman, and it took a lot of persuading to get her local IVF team to take her on:

I was the first single person to be treated at the hospital, but I think they're all changing now. They're thinking that single people do have a right as well. Where there's no father involved, they counsel you to make sure that if you do have a baby you are financially and emotionally fit to bring it up on your own.

Personal recommendation and reputation

If you know someone who has had IVF who can recommend a clinic, that is going to be helpful, and may be a big factor in helping you choose. However, you do need to remember that the nature of their fertility problem may be very different from your own, and it doesn't automatically follow that what has worked for someone else is going to be the best choice for you.

Now that so many people discuss fertility problems and treatments online, you may find a lot of Internet chatter about the relative merits of different centres. Some clinics do build up a good reputation among patients or among the medical profession, but patients and doctors often have different opinions about what makes an excellent fertility clinic. Patients may favour high success rates and new cutting-edge treatments, whereas medical professionals often respect clinics run by renowned teams who are carrying out valuable research, and these clinics will not always top the league tables when it comes to success rates.

Alison has been to a few different clinics during her treatment, and says she'd advise getting as much information from others as you can:

When I started out I didn't have anyone to talk to, or turn to. Nowadays if I was doing it, I'd be on all the blogs, all the

websites and all the forums searching for people's opinions.
I wish I'd spent more time checking clinics out.

You may want to use this quick checklist to make sure
you have taken into consideration the relevant issues
for you.

Checklist for choosing a clinic

- How close is the clinic to your home and/or
  workplace?
- Does it offer the treatment you need?
- Will you be eligible for treatment there?
- What are the clinic success rates for someone of
  your age?
- Is there a waiting list, and if so, how long is it?
- How much will your treatment cost?
- Did you like the atmosphere at the clinic?
- Do you know anyone else who has been treated
  there who might recommend it?
- Can the clinic offer early morning appointments if
  you need them?
- Does the staff have any particular expertise in rele-
  vant fields for you and/or your partner?
- Are you happy with the counselling and support
  offered to patients?

Choosing a clinic overseas

Traditionally, location may have been one of the most
important factors in choosing a clinic, but now more and
more people are choosing to travel overseas for fertility

treatment. This may be to access treatment they can't get at home, to get cheaper treatment or to avoid certain rules and regulations about IVF in their own countries. One common reason for travelling overseas is the relative availability of donated eggs and sperm, as some countries have shorter waiting lists for donor treatment than others.

Anyone who is considering travelling abroad for treatment should do their homework first. Different countries have different regulatory systems when it comes to fertility treatment, and it is important to make sure you are aware of the rules. You should also find out as much as you possibly can about the clinic you are planning to visit. This is particularly important if you are planning to use donor eggs or sperm, as the rules on donor anonymity vary. In some places, such as the UK, Sweden and New Zealand, all children born as a result of donor treatment will be able to trace their donor when they are older, but in some other countries the process remains totally anonymous.

If you're going to use a surrogate for your IVF and plan to do that overseas, you should consult a lawyer before you start, as surrogacy laws can be complex. Overseas clinics may not offer the relevant counselling (see Chapter 9) that covers the implications of using donor eggs or sperm, or a surrogate, and it would be advisable to seek this out at home first if you are not going to get the opportunity to talk things through with a counsellor otherwise.

You may find a clinic at home that has links with an overseas unit. When there are shortages of eggs or sperm, clinics sometimes link up with other centres abroad so that you can get access to treatment more quickly and easily. If this is the case, you may feel more confident that your own clinic has already done a lot of the checks as far as the overseas clinic is concerned. This may make the prospect of overseas treatment less daunting, but it will usually make it more expensive, too.

On a purely practical level, you should check that you will be able to get to the clinic at short notice if necessary, and that you will be able to find somewhere to stay when you get there. You should also be sure that you can contact the clinic easily from home. Communication with overseas clinics is often carried out by email, and although this can work well, it may be frustrating if you don't get quick replies to urgent queries. You will want to be sure there are always English-speaking members of staff on duty, and that any paperwork you need to sign is available in translation. The most frequent problems experienced by those who have treatment overseas are to do with language and communication.

If you are going to have your scans and blood tests carried out in a clinic at home, and only plan to travel for egg collection and embryo transfer, you will have to find a local clinic willing to do this. You should be clear how the results of tests and scans are going to be passed on to the overseas clinic. Although some clinics offer this service for people who are travelling overseas, others have understandable concerns about getting involved in treatment they don't have any control over. One fertility nurse I spoke to said she worried about the lack of support offered to patients: 'With a clinic at home, you know you are going to be well supported by the team treating you because you will have built up a relationship. It is just the sheer geography of going abroad that might make that really tricky. You will feel very vulnerable.'

Debbie carried on using the same clinic at home when she went abroad for donor treatment, and she found this reassuring:

> It was nice to know I had support in this country if I had a reaction to the medications I was taking, that there was somebody just a few hours away. I looked to my consultant here for initial advice about everything. I know people who haven't been able to find clinics that have supported them and you're forced to be on your own, which is really hard.

Perhaps unexpectedly, people sometimes find that going for treatment overseas can be less demanding than having treatment at home, as you can detach the process from your day-to-day life. This was one of the things Nicola was looking forward to about going to Spain for IVF treatment: 'Before, we've fitted IVF in around work, but this is an opportunity to turn it into a bit of a holiday and have a week off. We will relax, unwind a bit, and it will be an easier process than doing it at home.'

Although many people find it a positive experience, you will not necessarily be familiar with the culture of the country you are visiting. Furthermore, language and communication problems, or differences of attitude and manners, may be harder to deal with when you are already feeling vulnerable. You may be talking through a translator to the medical staff treating you, which can be awkward, and having tests and scans done at a clinic at home and the bulk of your treatment overseas can also lead to misunderstandings and misinterpretations. If you go into it aware of these potential problems, you are more likely to be able to avoid the pitfalls.

Types of treatment

You probably have some idea of what IVF involves, but once you get to the clinic, you may find there are other strange-sounding variations of treatment on offer, and lots of confusing acronyms: ICSI, IVM, PGS or PGD . . . It can be hard to know what's what, and what is best for you, so I've listed some of the main types of treatment you may come across in order to try to help you through the maze.

IVF

In a standard IVF cycle, a woman is given drugs to make her ovaries produce a number of eggs. These eggs are collected, and mixed with her partner's sperm in the laboratory, where they are left to fertilise. If embryos are produced, they can then be transferred to the womb, or frozen for future use.

ICSI

You may be more familiar with intra-cytoplasmic sperm injection, or ICSI, than you think, as television and newspaper reporters often use images of ICSI to illustrate all kinds of stories about infertility. You've probably seen them: those pictures of a hollow needle being pushed right into an egg are an illustration of ICSI, rather than normal IVF.

ICSI was developed in the early 1990s. It is used primarily to overcome male fertility problems, and has become extremely popular. During ICSI, the best sperm from the semen sample are selected by the embryologist, and injected straight into the woman's egg. This allows embryologists to use sperm that might not have been capable of breaking into an egg and fertilising it by themselves. ICSI has been a huge step forward in the treatment of male infertility, as prior to this many men with fertility problems would never have been able to have their own genetic children.

ICSI has been so successful that some clinics carry out as many, if not more, cycles of ICSI as of IVF. It may even be suggested by a clinic when there isn't a male fertility problem at all, purely because some doctors feel it can offer higher success rates, although clinical trials suggest this isn't actually the case. Obviously, there is more interference with the natural process of fertilisation when the sperm are injected right into the egg, and this is something you may want to take into consideration if you are being offered ICSI when there are no male factor problems to make it a necessity.

GIFT/ZIFT

These are variations of IVF that are rarely carried out now, although GIFT, gamete intra-fallopian transfer, was popular for a while in some clinics. A GIFT cycle starts out in the same way as IVF, but once the eggs have been collected they are returned to the fallopian tube with the partner's sperm, rather than being left in the laboratory to fertilise. In ZIFT, or zygote intra-fallopian transfer, the eggs are fertilised in the lab and then any resulting embryos are returned to the fallopian tube.

Natural-cycle IVF

It is possible to carry out the IVF procedures in a natural cycle, without using drugs to stimulate the ovaries and make them produce lots of eggs. It is much cheaper than traditional IVF as there is no drugs bill, and there is no danger of over-stimulating the ovaries (page 84), but success rates are inevitably much lower as there is only one egg for the embryologists to work with.

Soft, or mild, IVF

There is growing interest among many professionals in the idea of performing a gentler form of IVF, known as soft, or mild, IVF. Lower doses of the drugs are used, so the ovaries don't produce as many eggs, and it doesn't involve as much disruption to the woman's body. This reduces the risk of ovarian hyperstimulation syndrome (OHSS) (page 84), a common and potentially dangerous side effect of standard IVF. Those in favour of soft IVF note that it is also cheaper, as fewer drugs are involved, and you don't need as many injections, or as many visits to the clinic, making it feel far less intrusive.

IVM

In vitro maturation, or IVM, is a relatively new technique that involves taking eggs direct from the ovary when they are still immature. They are left to develop in the laboratory, and then mixed with sperm when they are ripe for fertilisation. Although you may need to take some drugs if you are having IVM, these will not be as disruptive as those used during IVF and you don't have the same risk of hyperstimulation. However, IVM relies on a woman having lots of immature eggs, known as resting follicles, in her ovaries. Only younger women, or those who have polycystic ovaries (page 10), are likely to have sufficient numbers to make carrying out IVM worthwhile.

PGD

Pre-implantation genetic diagnosis, or PGD, is used to test for known inherited conditions. If a couple know that they risk passing a condition on to future generations, they may choose to have PGD after suitable counselling. They will go through a normal IVF cycle, and once embryos are produced, they can then be tested to see whether they carry the conditions. In order to do this, one or two cells are extracted from an embryo that has divided into eight cells. The cells are tested, and only embryos that are clear will be replaced. PGD can be used to test for a fairly wide range of inherited conditions such as cystic fibrosis, muscular dystrophy, haemophilia and sickle-cell anaemia.

PGS

Pre-implantation genetic screening, or PGS, is a more recent adaptation of PGD used to check embryos for chromosomal abnormalities that it is thought may cause miscarriage or prevent embryos implanting. It is some-times recommended for older women, who are more at risk of having a child with chromosomal problems, or for those who have had recurrent miscarriages or repeated unsuccessful treatment cycles.

The checking of the embryos is carried out in exactly the same way as it is in PGD, by making a hole in the embryo and taking out a cell to test. PGS may be referred to as aneuploidy screening, and some clinics had seen it as an exciting new development in helping older women or those who had been unsuccessful with IVF in the past. In fact, research has shown that PGS is not always accurate. Some embryos contain a mixture of normal and abnormal cells, so extracting one to test can give a false result. Despite claims that it increases the IVF pregnancy rate by reducing the miscarriage risk, most of the evidence seems to suggest that pregnancy rates are actually lower after PGS, and more research is needed in this area.

Surgical sperm retrieval – PESA, MESA, TESE

Some men do not have sperm in their semen, although they ejaculate normally. This can occur if the tube that carries sperm from the testicles is blocked, or hasn't developed properly. Sometimes there may be a problem with sperm production. Men who have had a vasectomy reversal may find they still do not have any sperm in their ejaculate, as it is not always possible to mend a tube that has been cut or clipped.

It may be possible in such cases to retrieve the sperm surgically. Most men have some sperm in the epididymis (the coiled tubes at the top of the testicles where sperm are stored) or in the testicles themselves, even if they are immature sperm. If sperm are found, samples taken from surgical retrieval are usually frozen before being used in the future for ICSI. There are a number of different ways to retrieve sperm.

Percutaneous sperm aspiration, or PESA, involves using a fine needle to suck out some fluid from the epididymis. It is generally the first-choice method when it comes to surgical sperm retrieval, as it is fairly quick and there is no need to cut the scrotum or testicles.

Micro-epididymal sperm aspiration, or MESA, involves cutting through the scrotum and then inserting a needle into the epididymis to try to find sperm.

Testicular sperm extraction, or TESE, is used when it is not possible to get sperm from the epididymis. TESE involves making one or more small cuts in the testicles in order to take out a sample of tissue. The tissue will then be taken to the lab, so that the embryologists can see whether it contains any sperm.

The success of surgical sperm retrieval is not just dependent on the medical team carrying out the process, but also on the skills of the embryologists in the lab who face the often laborious search for viable sperm in the samples. The determination of a good embryologist to find moving sperm in such samples is impressive, and illustrates the care and dedication needed for this job. In some cases, it can take hours before a sperm they can use is found. When I spent time in the laboratory, I was able to watch on a screen as the embryologist beside me searched through a TESE sample for moving sperm. It was full of lumps of debris, and although there were sperm present, most were bent or misshapen, and showed few signs of life. Occasionally the embryologist would spot a sluggish sperm moving slowly forward and would track it before carefully knocking off the tail and sucking it into the ICSI pipette ready to be injected into an egg.

Assisted hatching

If you've had repeatedly unsuccessful IVF attempts, or you are at the top of the age range for fertility treatment at your clinic, doctors may suggest you consider assisted hatching. It is a procedure that isn't used often nowadays, as there is no clear evidence that it works. It involves thinning the outer layer of the embryo, or making a tiny hole in it, before replacing it in the womb during an IVF cycle.

Frozen embryo transfer

Women often produce more eggs than they are going to use in one cycle when they have IVF treatment, and if the eggs fertilise and there are good quality spare embryos, they can be frozen and returned to the womb in a later treatment cycle. Not all embryos survive the freezing and thawing process, and success rates are sometimes lower for frozen embryo transfers, but going through a frozen embryo cycle is far less invasive. There won't be as many visits to the clinic or as many drugs, and it is also much cheaper.

The next step

Now you know more about the types of treatment clinics may offer, and have an idea of what to look for when you are choosing a clinic, you should feel more confident about making your decisions. It will be an unfamiliar world, and it is easy to feel rather overwhelmed, but the next few chapters will guide you through the process from the very first appointment, so that you know what to expect during your treatment cycle.

Chapter three

Your First Appointment at the Clinic

You may experience a whole mix of emotions when you find yourself inside a fertility clinic as a patient for the first time. There can be a huge sense of relief that finally you are moving forward and taking some positive action, or a sense of gloom at the reality of having to accept that you are not going to get pregnant without medical help. For many of us who have to have fertility treatment, attending the IVF clinic is our first experience of being a regular hospital patient, and it may all seem rather strange at first.

Most people understandably feel nervous the first time they visit the clinic, and this chapter will explain what you might expect to find and who you might meet when you step through the clinic doors.

The clinic

Many fertility clinics run as units within larger hospitals, sometimes situated in the gynaecology or women's health departments. Others operate completely independently as stand-alone fertility centres. The differences between these ways of working are not likely to be particularly relevant to you as a patient, although the atmosphere in a large hospital will clearly not be the same as in a small independent clinic.

In larger hospitals the fertility unit is often part of a women's health or gynaecology department and that can mean that you are constantly finding yourself face to face with pregnant women. It is something you may want to bear in mind if you have a choice of clinics. I went to one hospital fertility unit recently and found myself sharing the lift with a woman in labour, which has the potential to be upsetting for anyone trying unsuccessfully to get pregnant. Jo's clinic was in the women's section of a hospital, and she says this made it quite hard at times: 'There were always pregnant women with huge bellies waddling around, and women going in for early pregnancy scans. They'd have kids with them sometimes, and I know it wasn't their fault, but it felt as if they were rubbing it in.'

The size of a fertility clinic can vary greatly, with some starting dozens of IVF treatment cycles every day, and others carrying out only a few every month. The staffing levels will depend on the workload, and some clinics offer a wider variety of treatment options than others. The physical environment can also differ greatly, but this shouldn't be taken as a measure of the level of care you will receive, or of the relative chances of getting pregnant – the aesthetics may make a difference to the way you feel about the place, but they are not an indicator of success.

The waiting room

You are going to spend far more time than you would ever have expected or wanted to in the clinic waiting room. It's the first place you'll see in the clinic, and most of us end up making some kind of judgement about the clinic as a whole based on how we felt when we first walked into the waiting room.

I've spent time in dozens of clinic waiting rooms, and there's something about the atmosphere that is unique. No one wants to find themselves in a fertility clinic, and the stigma still attached to infertility means that most of us look as uncomfortable as we feel. There's rarely any sense of camaraderie, and people often try to avoid eye contact, let alone striking up a conversation with one another. I had IVF treatment on and off over a period of six years, often visiting the clinic two or three times a week, and yet in all that time I only once ended up chatting to another patient, and I have to admit that was because she spoke to me first. I wasn't the only one to feel that way. Isobel admits she really disliked spending time in the waiting room at her clinic:

> You sit there in the waiting room and nobody speaks to anybody. It should be the first time you can actually be open. You're surrounded by people who are in the same position and probably feel the same as you, but it was just awful, like you didn't want to admit you were actually there.

The waiting rooms often have a similar look: pastel-coloured walls or furnishings, sofas if you're lucky, uncomfortable plastic chairs if you're not, and perhaps a coffee table with some well-thumbed women's magazines or leaflets about support groups and sexually transmitted infections. Some have a radio crackling away in the background, others may have a TV tuned into daytime programmes. You may get a water fountain or a coffee machine, and for some reason nearly all the waiting rooms I've been to contain at least one potted plant, often slightly wilted and past its best.

Even in the most efficient clinics, you may find that appointments don't always keep to time, and waiting times can range from minutes to hours. I regularly sat for an hour or so in the waiting room after my allotted appointment time, and even if you take some work to do, or a book to read, it can be hard to concentrate when you are waiting for results, or to find out how things are going with your treatment. It is frustrating if you're stuck in the waiting room for a lengthy period: you don't want to be there in the first place, there are a million and one other things you ought to be doing, you may have lied at work about where you are and you're certainly going to have difficulty explaining where you've been when you get back. By the time you get in to see the doctor, you may be feeling thoroughly fed up. If this happens, try to remember that often you're waiting because staff are busy dealing with other patients. Appointments can overrun if things don't go according to plan, or a patient breaks down in floods of tears after an unexpected test result. Staff will need to take time to sort things out and they can't just usher patients out of the clinic because they've gone over their allocated time. If you encounter problems during your treatment, you would expect the staff to take time to help, and running overtime can be an indication of a clinic where they are doing just that.

The consulting room

Once you finally make it out of the waiting room, the next place in the clinic you are likely to find yourself is the consulting room, where you will have appointments with the consultant, doctor or nurse. The consulting rooms at clinics are generally fairly similar to your local doctor's surgery with a desk, often piled high with files and papers, a computer and chairs. There is usually a bed for examinations behind a flimsy curtain and sometimes an ultrasound scanner if scans are carried out in the consulting room, although some clinics have a separate scanning room.

The men's room

When we had our first cycle of IVF, it wasn't uncommon for men to be asked to use the men's toilets when they had to produce a sperm sample, but now most clinics have a special room for the purpose. Over the years, I've heard a number of horror stories from men about the places they were expected to make do – from hospital toilets that had doors with huge gaps above and below them, to the clinic where the key to the men's room was attached to a piece of yellow plank that the men had to carry with them when they went off to give a sample, which seemed guaranteed to make them feel as conspicuous as possible.

Doctors are aware of the need to make it all a bit easier, although exactly what you get by way of a men's room depends on the clinic. Sometimes it may be little more than a rather stark, small room with a sink in the corner, and a few dog-eared ·magazines, whereas other clinics invest in DVDs. It is not ideal, or remotely romantic, but they are trying.

The operating theatre

You won't usually get as far as the operating theatre until it's time for egg collection, but most clinics have their own facilities for this. The operating theatre is used when eggs are collected and embryos replaced, and for other invasive techniques, such as surgical sperm collection. There is usually a hospital bed in the centre of the room surrounded by medical equipment. It can all look a bit alarming, but most of the procedures carried out in the fertility clinic operating theatre are straightforward and routine.

The laboratory

As the scientists in the laboratory work closely with the medical team during egg collections and embryo transfers, the lab is often connected to the operating theatre and may open out into it. Eggs, sperm and embryos are kept in the laboratory in incubators to ensure they stay at the right temperature. Frozen eggs, sperm and embryos are stored in special straws inside large churn-like buckets. There are microscopes and equipment for viewing and inseminating, and for preparing eggs and sperm.

The laboratory is carefully maintained at a set temperature and it is a very clean, sterile environment. As a patient you are unlikely to see any more of it than a glimpse through the open door. When we first started fertility treatment, we were invited in to the laboratory to peer down a microscope to get a look at our embryos, but this is no longer standard practice and when patients get to see their embryos it is usually on a screen. Staff have to change into special clothes and shoes before they are allowed to enter the lab in order to protect the eggs, sperm and embryos.

The counselling room

Some larger clinics that have a counsellor on site have a room designated for counselling. This usually seems to be the tiniest room in the building, and there may just be a couple of chairs and a table.

The clinic staff

Who you meet at any given time during your treatment will depend on the way your clinic does things, on staffing levels and also your individual circumstances. However, there are a number of key staff members you will come across. Each will play a different role in the IVF process, and you may see them at different stages of your treatment, but as one consultant explains, the ability to work together as integral parts of one unit is essential in a fertility clinic: 'When patients come to see us, they don't see us as individual practitioners. They see the IVF team providing care, and so it has to be a team effort. It's very different from going to see a surgeon or physician to solve your chest problem or cardiological problem.'

The receptionist

When you arrive at the clinic, the receptionist is likely to be the first person you'll talk to. They'll probably be the one to greet you every time you visit, and may answer the phone when you call as well. The receptionist is the gateway to the clinic, and they nearly always seem to be incredibly friendly and sympathetic people, although I daresay there's an absolute dragon lurking behind the reception desk at a fertility clinic somewhere in the world. In a small clinic, you'll probably get to know the receptionist quite well, whereas a larger clinic may have a team of receptionists.

The doctors

Some clinics are run by one consultant, others will have a whole team of consultants and doctors. The doctors and consultants will have completed a general training in medicine first, followed by some specialist training in fertility. The consultants tend to lead the team, but how much you see of them varies from clinic to clinic. At some places, they will conduct the initial consultations with patients and carry out the procedures in the operating theatre, but at others you may end up seeing a consultant only if there is some kind of complication or difficulty.

All doctors will have a broad knowledge of infertility, and will be familiar with the conditions that can cause problems and how to treat them. Some may also specialise in particular areas of infertility, and they may spend part of their time doing research in their specialist field. Consultants working in larger hospitals may sometimes carry out general obstetric and gynaecology work alongside their fertility clinics, others may do clinical or scientific research or specialist surgery, and their daily routine can vary hugely, depending on both their specialist interest and where they work.

Patients can feel rather intimidated by the consultants and doctors. They seem to hold the key to the thing you most want, which can make them appear all-powerful. Many consultants are wonderfully warm, understanding and sympathetic characters, but others can sometimes be guilty of playing up to their status, and you shouldn't let this make you feel uncomfortable about asking questions and getting all the information you need.

Debbie admits that she sometimes found it difficult to make sure she asked everything she wanted to at the clinic, and this is a common feeling: 'I'm not a very assertive person, and I find myself going into complete patient mode when I am at the clinic. Afterwards I'd think, *I should have asked that*, or *I should have said that. I should have been more assertive.*'

The nurses

Most fertility nurses will have started with a general nursing training, and may have specialised in another area of women's health, such as midwifery or gynaecology before moving into fertility. There are a range of nursing courses they can take that are geared towards reproductive health, and some will specialise further once they've gone into the fertility field, by perhaps running egg-donation programmes or managing units.

The nurses work with the doctors, but the degree of responsibility they take can vary. In some clinics, the nurses have a similar role to the more senior doctors, carrying out all the medical procedures such as egg collection, embryo transfers and even surgical sperm retrieval. You may see them for consultations during IVF, and they may train the junior doctors in the unit. In these clinics, you will probably see a doctor only if there is a problem. In other clinics, the nurses may play a more traditional role and will be taking blood, giving injections and assisting the doctors, and they will spend more time with the patients.

If nurses at the unit you visit take on more responsibility, you shouldn't feel you are short-changed by seeing them rather than a doctor. One nurse I spoke to was clear that it might not always be in a patient's best interest to insist on seeing a doctor:

> We tend to say to people, if you haven't seen a doctor, that's because everything is OK. There is still that perception that I've paid five thousand pounds, so I want to see the doctor. It's a shame, as there may be a nurse who is more competent and better skilled.

It is usually the nurses that you will see most at the clinic, and they may be the people you find yourself turning to with any questions or problems. The nurses often take on a counselling role, too, as people sometimes find it is easier to discuss any problems as they arise with the nurse, rather than waiting for a session with the counsellor.

The embryologists

The scientists who support the medical team and look after the eggs, sperm and embryos are embryologists. They are the people you may spot around the clinic dressed as if they've just emerged from an operating theatre, wearing what look like shower caps.

They will usually have taken a science-based degree and then carried on with specialist training in embryology. Embryology has become a popular and highly competitive area, as it allows scientists to use their skills in an exciting and rapidly changing and developing field, while also being able to see the results of that work for real people on a daily basis.

The embryologists work in the clinic laboratory, carrying out any procedures needed to prepare the eggs and sperm, and to help fertilisation. They take care of any resulting embryos until they are ready to be returned to the woman's womb. They are also responsible for freezing spare embryos, for keeping them safely stored and thawing them when they are going to be used, as well as freezing eggs and sperm.

The amount of contact you have with the embryology team varies from clinic to clinic. Sometimes you may not meet them at all, and they are shadowy figures who you only see coming and going from the laboratory. At other clinics, the embryologists will come and talk to you about your eggs and sperm, and will be responsible for keeping you updated about fertilisation rates and the progress of any resulting embryos.

Andrologists and seminologists

Some larger clinics may have male-fertility specialists working on the team. Andrology is the male equivalent of gynaecology, and a consultant andrologist is a doctor who specialises in the causes and treatment of male infertility.

In larger hospitals, there may be a team of seminologists, especially if there is a sperm bank. Like embryologists, the seminologists will have a science-based degree and they work in a laboratory. They only deal with sperm, and will be responsible for semen analysis, freezing and storing.

Administrative staff

Larger clinics will also have administrative staff, as IVF creates lots of paperwork and records that need keeping up to date. Arranging appointments, scheduling diaries and looking after the day-to-day operation of the clinic is a huge task. You may never see the admin staff, but their backup is crucial to keep things running smoothly.

Your first appointment

The initial appointment at the fertility clinic is usually with a member of the medical team, most often a consultant or doctor, but sometimes a nurse. The aim of this appointment is to make sure the fertility clinic staff are fully aware of your situation in order to work out the most appropriate way to proceed with treatment, assuming that it is necessary.

At this appointment, the doctor or nurse will want to know about your medical history. For a woman, this will include questions about your age, weight and menstrual-cycle pattern. For both partners, it will be important to find out about any previous surgery, serious illnesses and sexually transmitted infections that could affect your fertility.

Most clinics like to do a physical examination of both partners, but it is usually just a simple check to make sure everything is where it ought to be. For the man, this will mean ensuring there are no obvious problems with the testicles, or with the tubes that carry the sperm away from them. For the woman, there may be an internal examination and possibly a smear test and a vaginal ultrasound scan, too. If you're considering IVF, the chances are that you will be only too familiar with vaginal ultrasound scans, but if for some reason you haven't had one before, this is a straightforward process. The doctor, or nurse, inserts a probe into the vagina and uses ultrasound to check that the womb and ovaries look normal. The scan works by using sound waves that send out echoes as they bounce off your body, and these are used to give a picture. You will usually be able to see this on a screen, although it is difficult to work out what is what if you aren't an expert. The scan is a bit like a painless cervical smear test. You will have a number of scans during IVF treatment, and although initially the procedure may seem a little odd and rather undignified, it will soon become routine.

It is particularly useful if you can make sure the clinic has the medical records of all the previous investigations, tests and treatments you've had for your fertility problem. Sometimes, when people change clinics, they are reluctant to let their original clinic know that they are moving on, and don't like to ask for their records. In fact, it is common for people to move from one clinic to another, and it will save a lot of time if your new clinic has access to up-to-date medical records.

What happens next depends on how far down the line you already are with testing and treatment. Sometimes, the clinic may want to send you for additional tests you haven't had, or they may want to repeat some tests for themselves, particularly semen analysis.

Many couples feel incredibly nervous about their first appointment. This is perfectly normal, and doctors and nurses recognise that this can be a difficult time. It may be particularly upsetting if they are going to have to tell you at this point that some form of assisted conception may be the only way that you will be able to conceive. One consultant I spoke to said staff were aware that for many patients just coming in to the clinic could feel quite traumatic: 'I'm sure for some people when they come in it is a shock, and I think everybody is nervous. Just walking into the hospital, even if you're not outwardly nervous, you will feel apprehensive inside, and the nursing staff support the patients from when they first come in.'

By the end of the appointment, you should have some idea of the way ahead. The clinic may want to carry out more investigations in order to be certain why you aren't managing to conceive naturally, or you may be ready to move on to treatment fairly quickly although there will still be some preparation before you begin.

Chapter four

Before You Start Treatment

Once both you and your doctor have decided that IVF seems to be the most likely way ahead for you, there may be a number of tests and checks to be carried out before you can start. I was surprised that there were more of these at this late stage, and you may feel as if this is yet another hurdle that will slow things down, but it ensures the medical team have all the information they need before you go ahead.

Tests

You may have to have some new tests before you start treatment, and the clinic may also want to repeat tests you've had done before, especially if they were originally carried out some time ago. I've listed the most common tests overleaf.

Rubella

For women, there will be a blood test to check rubella immunity. Rubella, or German measles, can be dangerous in early pregnancy, putting babies at risk of deafness, blindness and learning difficulties. If you are not immune, you will need a rubella vaccination before you start treatment.

Hepatitis B and C

There are different varieties of hepatitis, which is caused by a virus and affects the liver. It does not always have any obvious symptoms and the fertility clinic may want to carry out a blood test for hepatitis B or hepatitis C for both partners. The chances of passing the infection on to a baby during a normal pregnancy are not high, but hepatitis is infectious, and staff and other patients could be at risk if proper procedures are not put in place. Not all clinics will treat patients who test positive for hepatitis, and some will not freeze embryos in these circumstances. If this is the case, they should be able to refer you to another unit where they are equipped to help patients who have had a positive hepatitis test result.

HIV

It is quite usual to do an HIV test before going ahead with IVF. As with hepatitis, the risk of passing on the HIV virus to a child during pregnancy is low, especially if there is prior knowledge of the condition, but not many clinics have the facilities to treat HIV-positive patients. It is still possible to get treatment if you are HIV-positive, but you may need to travel to a clinic that is set up to handle blood-borne infections.

Semen analysis

Most clinics want to carry out their own semen analysis before starting IVF. Sometimes this can be done at home if you live close to the clinic, but often you will be asked to produce a sample in the men's room at the clinic. Sperm samples deteriorate if they don't get to the laboratory quickly, and should not be exposed to extreme temperatures, as this seminologist explains:

> They have to get the sample to us within an hour of it being produced. If it's a freezing cold day in the middle of winter, I usually tell them to put it in their trouser pockets or something like that. We've had people put samples on the car radiator to keep them warm, or put them in the fridge overnight, but you shouldn't do this, as extremes of temperature can definitely do damage.

The clinic may do a sperm antibody test at this stage, too, as this can affect the way the sperm function and stop them fertilising an egg.

Ovarian reserve testing

Many clinics like to test how many immature eggs are in your ovaries (known as your ovarian reserve) before you start treatment, in order to assess how you might respond to the drugs given during IVF. There is some debate among fertility specialists about how valid these tests are.

There are a number of different methods used to check ovarian reserve. Traditionally, doctors have usually looked at levels of FSH, or follicle-stimulating hormone, which helps the eggs grow in the ovaries. They may also look at levels of LH, or luteinising hormone, oestrodial, inhibin B and AMH (or anti-Mullerian hormone), all of which can give an indication of how many immature eggs there are. Some clinics may also carry out an antral follicle count, which involves looking at the numbers of the tiny follicles in the ovary in their early stages of development.

Of all of these tests, AMH is now generally considered to be one of the most reliable, as it can be carried out at any time during the monthly cycle and doesn't tend to fluctuate much, unlike FSH which can vary from cycle to cycle. Some doctors question the value of any ovarian reserve testing, as they believe your age is a more reliable indicator of whether treatment is likely to be successful. In a younger woman, a result showing a low ovarian reserve can indicate a problem, but in an older woman, age is more relevant. It is thought ovarian reserve testing probably gives a picture of the *number* of eggs left in the ovaries, whereas the *quality* of the eggs is more dependent on age.

If tests suggest you have a very low ovarian reserve, some clinics may suggest that you should consider egg dona-tion immediately, but others prefer to see how your body responds to the drugs before going down this path. IVF can be successful when ovarian reserve tests are poor, but this is something you should discuss with your doctor.

Full blood count

The results of a full blood count give an indication of your general health, so this is sometimes carried out at the same time to alert the medical team to any other problems.

Sexually transmitted infection tests

Clinics may also want to test both partners for chlamydia, gonorrhoea and/or syphilis, as you can have these sexually transmitted infections without necessarily being aware of them, and they can have a devastating effect on your fertility.

CMV-status testing

If you are going to be using donated eggs or sperm, you will usually have a test for cytomegalorvirus, or CMV. You've probably never heard of it, but CMV is a very common infection, and it is thought that at least half of us will have had it during our lifetime without knowing it. Once you have been infected, the antibodies remain in your body forever, and will show positive in tests. Doctors may prefer not to give eggs or sperm from a CMV-positive donor to a recipient who has never had the virus, and this is why the test is carried out. This is really just a precautionary measure, as CMV does not usually cause any problems.

Ultrasound scan

You will usually have an ultrasound scan before you start treatment, to make sure that there are not any fibroids (page 12) or polyps (lumps of tissue) in the womb that could prevent implantation. The scan also gives a clear view of the ovaries. If the medical team want to check your ovarian reserve using an antral follicle count, this is done during the ultrasound scan.

Trial embryo transfer

In the final stage of treatment, the team will hope to be transferring one or two embryos that have been fertilised in the laboratory back into your womb. This is done by inserting a catheter into the vagina, which passes into the womb itself through the cervix.

I'd always imagined the cervix to go in a straight line from the vagina to the womb, but apparently the path can be quite awkward, and the length of the cervix varies. Doctors often like to do a practice run either before you start treatment, or when you have your eggs collected, to highlight any problems, as this head of clinic explains: 'We do a mock embryo transfer at egg collection, because if you do it in advance you know the route. You think of the cervix as a tube, but actually it has branches all over the place. They are all different sizes, and can have kinks and blind alleys.'

The trial embryo transfer is a straightforward procedure, similar to a smear test, and means there's no risk of suddenly discovering you have a particularly difficult cervix to negotiate when your embryos are ready and waiting to be put in the womb.

Understanding your treatment

Most clinics arrange some kind of meeting where they will talk you through what happens during treatment, in order to give you an idea of what to expect. This may be part of a large open day, a meeting attended by a number of patients, or an individual session. If you do attend an open day or large meeting, you will probably have a personal chat with a doctor or nurse before you start anyway.

Don't be afraid to ask questions at these sessions,

and don't ever feel your question is too silly or too unimportant, or that it's something you should already know. These introductory meetings are aimed at making sure you have all the relevant information and helping you to understand as much as you can about the process, as the head of one clinic explained:

> We have an open day where patients are talked through assisted conception, and we have a session where they can ask individual questions and pick up literature. Once you break the ice, once somebody asks the first question, then everybody tends to start talking. They're all here for the same reason.

You will probably be given some leaflets, brochures or other documents about the treatment, and it is worth taking the time to sit down and read through these. Even if you take notes at an information meeting, there may be things you are unsure of afterwards. If you've picked up all the available literature, you may well find the answers to your questions.

Making sure that you are well informed can also help you feel more in control of what is happening, and reading books or going online may also be useful. People who have had IVF often say that one of the most helpful things is talking to others who have been through fertility treatment about their experiences, and there are lots of online forums where you can do this.

Kate is waiting to start her first IVF cycle, and she says she has got most of the information about her impending treatment from other patients:

I felt I was being an annoyance at the clinic. They need to be more considerate and remember that they do it every day but we don't. I felt you had to find out for yourself. There was nobody there telling you. The majority of the information I have got has come from other women who have been there, done that and got the T-shirt.

Your drugs regime

There are many different brands of IVF drugs on the market, and the drugs you are given will depend on your circumstances as well as the brands your clinic tends to use. You shouldn't worry if someone else you know is taking a different drug, or has been prescribed a different dosage.

We will go through the drugs you may be given and what they do in detail in the next chapter, but treatment tends to begin with some drugs to switch off your own hormones, a process known as down-regulation, although patients may miss out this phase of treatment, depending on what doctors feel is best. The other main drugs you will be taking are called gonadotrophins, they stimulate the ovaries to try to get them to produce a number of eggs. There will also be a drug to mature the eggs, which is usually given as a late-night injection, and some to support your body after the embryos have been transferred. You may find you are prescribed additional drugs during an IVF cycle, either because of your individual circumstances or because your clinic believes they are helpful.

Injecting

Most couples going through fertility treatment do their own injections, and it certainly makes it far easier if you are able to do it yourself. This often worries people before they start treatment, but one of the fertility nurses I spoke to assured me that most patients cope well when it comes to it:

We have ladies come through who swear blind they are needle-phobic, and then manage it no problem. We try to keep it as informal as possible and to reassure them before they see the needle that the anticipation is much worse than the actual injection. I guarantee that as soon as they've done it they're going to say it wasn't as bad as they thought it would be.

My husband did my injections, so I didn't ever get as far as finding out that it might not be as bad as I'd expected. Having your partner do this is a good way of involving him in the process. We were quite anxious about being sent home with a bag full of injection equipment and drugs, and left to do it ourselves, but it wasn't nearly as difficult as we'd anticipated.

In our first cycle, we did it the old-fashioned way, using a needle and syringe, but later we were given a self-injection kit. It is much easier, as you just put the kit, which looks a bit like a large pen, against your skin and press the button. There's a clicking noise as the spring inside releases the needle and it is propelled into the skin. Injecting at home for the first time can be unnerving, and if you suddenly feel you can't do it, or something goes wrong, call your clinic. The staff are used to dealing with these concerns, and will be able to help.

Even if the first time is difficult, most people quickly get used to the injections, and it becomes a matter of routine. Kylie says she was surprised how quickly this happened to her: 'When you get home and you have to do it for the first time, it is nerve-wracking, but you get past that. I suppose it's like driving. When you first start to drive it's nerve-wracking, but once you get the hang of it, it's just everyday life.'

Paperwork

There will be some paperwork before you start your treatment cycle, and it helps to ensure you have understood the treatment you are being offered, and that you have given your consent. You will also have to decide what you will do with any spare embryos that may be left over during treatment. You may want to freeze them for use in the future, to donate them to research or to another couple who need both donor eggs and sperm.

Work and your impending treatment cycle

Some women manage to work all the way through their IVF treatment without any real problems, but others end up either taking some time off, cutting down on their working hours or even giving up work for a while. The two main factors affecting this are your employer and your clinic.

If your clinic is close to either your home or your office, it is going to be far less disruptive than having long journeys that take you out of your way every time you have an appointment. Some clinics open early in the morning for scans during treatment, so that women can go before work. Staff are increasingly aware of the problems patients face trying to fit their treatment around work, as this consultant explains:

> We see patients before they go to work in the morning so it is not disruptive to their working day. We try to make it less disruptive wherever we can because all of those things make a difference. If you think about it for yourself, how would you manage it? I couldn't do IVF – I could never get away from here to go off and have my appointments.

The other factor that comes into play here is the number of appointments you have during your cycle. This differs from clinic to clinic, and may depend on your response to the drugs, too. Discuss it with the clinic before you start, as that will give you some idea of what to expect.

The level of freedom you have at work will make a difference. If your hours are flexible, and you can make up for any lost time at a later date, you may manage to fit clinic appointments around work. For those working more rigid hours, however, or in jobs where they cannot easily disappear for a few hours now and again, it is more difficult, as this nurse explains: 'Generally most people don't have brilliant support from work, so it is kept a secret, and that secret is an enormous burden. Teachers are probably one of the most stressed groups that come through. They really struggle because they are always trying to do it in the holidays.'

Some companies have enlightened policies on fertility treatment, and will allow you time off or unpaid leave as you need it, although these may still be in the minority. If you work for a large company that has a human resources department, you may want to check to see whether your employer has a policy on time off for fertility treatment.

There are employers who are extremely unsympathetic towards fertility treatment, and they may assume that you are less committed to your job if they know you're trying to have a baby. Not everyone feels able to be honest about it with their boss. In these circumstances it will help if you have a colleague you can trust, as confiding in them may mean they can cover for you if clinic appointments mean you are running late or have to leave early. If you need time off and you are worried that it will make things tough at work if you tell your employer, you can always see your doctor, who will usually be happy to sign you off work for a while during treatment.

Alison has had five IVF cycles, and says she feels there is very little understanding in the workplace: 'I wish companies would support people who have IVF. There is nothing that says you can have time off, and people don't talk about it. I have told all my bosses, and I don't think it has helped my career.'

Alison is not alone in thinking that this has had a negative impact on her career. Patients often say that they feel promotions and pay rises do not come their way because they have been honest about what they are doing, and because of the amount of time they've had to take off, but this can be hard to prove.

Women who intend to work throughout most of the cycle will still need to take a day off work when they have egg collection. Although you may have a rough idea when this will be, it isn't always easy to pinpoint, as it will depend on how you respond to the drugs. You will also need time off when you have the embryos transferred to your womb, and most people prefer to take the entire day off for this.

When we started IVF, I was working as a television journalist, which is not a particularly flexible job, and fitting in two or three appointments a week at the clinic wasn't easy. I hadn't told anyone at work about my treatment, and it got so awkward that I ended up having to take a week off to cover the last scans, egg collection and embryo transfer, and then went back to work after that. Having interviewed dozens of other women about their IVF over the years, I've realised that most people do it the other way round, and take time off after embryo transfer, preferring not to be at work for the two weeks between that and the pregnancy test. For me, it was the logistics of trying to fit clinic appointments around my job that was so difficult, and once I got into the waiting period after embryo transfer, I preferred to have the distractions of work. How you feel about this is a personal thing, and you may find that you change your mind once you actually start treatment, so be prepared for this and think about how you will deal with it if you do find you want to take some time off.

Telling other people

What you tell other people about your infertility and treatment, or whether you tell them at all, is a difficult decision. Some people are clear about it: either they don't want anyone to know, or they want it all out in the open and are happy to tell everyone. Most of us hover somewhere in the middle, telling just some of our friends and family.

There are certainly advantages to telling people. You don't get the endless questions about when you're going to get round to having children, or pressure about not leaving it too late. Your friends and family will try to be sympathetic and understanding. However, you have to accept that no one can fully appreciate what IVF is like unless they've been through it themselves. People may say things with the best possible motives that are very upsetting to you.

Toni told most of her friends and family when she was having treatment, and although on the whole she was pleased to have their support, she admits it wasn't always easy:

> I was quite open, and most friends and family knew what was going on. Sometimes it helped, but sometimes I found it a bit annoying. They're just concerned about what's going on, but it may have been better that they didn't know, although if things had gone wrong, I would have needed their support.

Everyone has an opinion about IVF, and with so much coverage of the issue in the media, people sometimes assume they know a lot about it. Your friends and family may not understand that fertility treatment doesn't always work, and it can be hard to have to deal with their expectations. This can be a particular problem if your treatment isn't successful, as they will all be waiting to find out whether it has worked. Having to go over the disappointment time and time again for all your friends and family can be very upsetting. One of the nurses I spoke to says she warns patients to think carefully before telling others:

> When people start fertility treatment, they get quite excited and want to go and tell people, but if you've only told a couple of close friends, then it is probably easier. I say, remember not to tell the world and his wife you are going through treatment, because if it doesn't work, you've got the world and his wife to tell.

Not telling anyone at all can cause problems, too. You may find yourself having to lie about things when it comes to frequent visits to the clinic, and your emotional state during treatment. Your decision about who to tell may be based on how much you see of your family and friends, and how much you feel you need to tell them at any given point. Najeeb and his partner told their families exactly what they were doing during their first cycle, but were more cautious when they tried again:

> They knew we were having IVF, but after the first cycle we didn't dwell on dates or specific times because we didn't want the phone calls to say, did you have a test today, how did you get on at the clinic, how many eggs did you get . . . We didn't want that added pressure. They are so desperate to have grandchildren that they are really worried, and we didn't want them to be upset for us at the bad times.

If you opt not to tell people about your cycle, you may still want to confide in one or two close friends or relatives, which means you will be able to get some support and have someone to talk to, without feeling everyone you know is sitting watching your progress through IVF from the sidelines. It may help to be slightly vague about exactly when you expect to be at each stage of your cycle if you are telling people about it, as this can give you some breathing space.

Ready for treatment

Now you've gone through all the preparation, you may start to feel quite excited, as things are finally about to get underway after what has often been a long and difficult route to IVF. We will now look at each stage of the treatment process in detail, to try to allay any worries or anxieties you may have.

Chapter five

Preparing the Eggs

The first part of the IVF treatment cycle centres on getting the ovaries to produce eggs that can then be collected and fertilised in the laboratory. During this time, the clinic's attention is focused on the woman, and the role of the male partner will be largely supportive until the eggs are collected. He will give his semen sample at that point, and the sperm will be prepared ready to inseminate the eggs.

The drugs regime

We have seen that there are three main stages of drug treatment during the IVF cycle: the down-regulation to turn off your hormones, the stimulation to produce the eggs, and then the final drug to mature the eggs. You might not use all of them, and you may take some additional drugs if your doctor thinks it will help in your individual circumstances.

Down-regulation

Most IVF cycles begin with a period of down-regulation. This switches off your normal hormones and allows the doctors to have greater control over your ovaries. The drugs used for this are either taken as a nasal spray or by injection. If you don't like injections, you may find it easier to use a nasal spray, although it does taste pretty vile.

The down-regulating drugs are usually started in the menstrual cycle before the month in which you are due to begin treatment. You will either be given a specific date to go back to the clinic, or asked to report back once your period has started. Most women take the down-regulating drugs for around two or three weeks, but the length of time varies.

There can be unpleasant menopausal side effects with these drugs, because they close down your hormones and induce a state similar to the menopause. You may have headaches, mood changes or hot flushes, and people often find this a difficult part of the IVF process. Emma had classic menopausal symptoms when she took the down-regulating drugs: 'I went through the hot flushes and night sweats associated with the menopause. I would literally wake up soaking wet, and I was up and down emotionally, and quite tearful.'

It is important not to worry unduly about side effects before you get to that point, as not everyone has problems with down-regulating drugs. Clare was well informed about possible problems, and was concerned that she didn't experience any of the things she was expecting: 'I've been through three down-regulations now, and I don't get the horrendous blinding headaches and mood swings and night sweats that some of my friends complained about. That actually worried me, because I thought if I wasn't getting any of the symptoms, I couldn't be down-regulating properly.'

Like Clare, I didn't have any menopausal symptoms, and my main problem was trying to remember to use my nasal spray regularly every four hours. Initially, it was fine as I was so keen to do everything right, but when I was a bit further into the process I would sometimes get so busy at work that I didn't notice the time, and ended up sniffing an hour late. Of course, that is not to be recommended, but it didn't do any harm.

In some cases, the clinic may suggest that you miss out this initial phase of down-regulation, and move straight onto the next part of the treatment cycle. This is known as a 'short protocol' and it speeds up the process considerably. However, it is not suitable for everyone, and not all clinics offer this.

The stimulating drugs

The next phase of the cycle involves stimulating the ovaries, and you will be injecting drugs to try to make your ovaries produce lots of eggs. In a natural cycle, many follicles start growing each month but only one becomes dominant and produces an egg. During IVF, the aim is to get more of the follicles to carry on growing, and to produce more than one egg.

The drugs used for this part of the cycle contain follicle-stimulating hormone, FSH, and some also contain luteinising hormone, LH. Originally, these drugs were made from the purified urine of menopausal women, as women of this age produce lots of FSH and LH, which is excreted in their urine. There were fantastic stories of lorries collecting nuns' urine, as convents were an obvious place to look when the manufacturers needed to find concentrations of women of a certain age to donate their urine. Nowadays, most of the drugs are produced in a more mundane way in the laboratory.

Most of us pay for the drugs ourselves, and the prices of different brands vary considerably. There is no evidence that the more expensive drugs produce better results or more pregnancies, but some clinics prefer certain brands and you should be led by your doctor on this. You may want to shop around a little if you are going to buy them yourself, as not all pharmacies charge the same price for a particular brand. Make sure you read the instructions, and refrigerate any drugs that need to be kept cold, as not storing them properly can make them less effective.

On the whole, people don't report physical side effects from these drugs, and it is the emotional impact that is more difficult to deal with. As the eggs grow, women often feel bloated. I always felt a bit like an over-ripe fruit, but these feelings don't normally kick in until the end of the cycle when you are close to egg collection. Lulu says she didn't notice any physical effects until the end of her IVF cycle: 'It was fine to start with, but I did get uncomfortable two or three days before the egg collection. I remember being in bed the day before because I was extremely bloated. It wasn't painful, just very uncomfortable.'

Scans and blood tests

The tests you have during the stimulating phase of the treatment cycle will vary. You may be asked to go in every day for scans and blood tests, or you may need to visit only two or three times. During this period, the drugs will be stimulating the follicles, and the clinic will be monitoring your response to make sure the eggs are collected at the right time.

Vaginal ultrasound scans will enable the team to see how your ovaries are responding to the drugs. Initially, there may not seem to be much happening, but as you go through the cycle, you may start to see on the scan a honeycomb of follicles around the ovary. The growing follicles are carefully monitored and measured at every scan. The exact size they have to reach before you have the injection to ripen them varies, but it is usually somewhere around the 18mm mark. Not all clinics do blood tests every time you have a scan, but they can be another useful check to see how your body is responding to the drugs. Depending on your response to the stimulation, the team may adjust the drugs you are taking – this doesn't indicate that something is wrong, just that the initial dosage might not have been right for your body.

During this stage of the cycle, women often find that they feel extremely emotional, and you may find yourself hanging on every word as the medical team carry out your scans. If things seem to be going well, you may find you are elated, but then feel yourself starting to worry again before the next scan. Each one can turn into another hurdle to be got over along the way. Things don't always go exactly according to plan, and sometimes cycles do have to be cancelled because the ovaries haven't responded to the drugs. This can be hugely disappointing, but it doesn't necessarily mean that another attempt won't be more successful.

hCG injection

The last injection is of hCG, or human chorionic gonadotrophin, and is given to ripen the eggs once they have reached a suitable size for harvesting; without it they would not mature. The timing of the injection is extremely important, as your egg collection must take place once a specific length of time has elapsed. The injection is usually done late at night so that the egg collection can be carried out around 36 hours later, which is first thing in the morning.

When we had our first IVF cycle, we had to have the hCG injection done at the hospital, possibly partly to make sure we didn't do it at the wrong time. It was an odd experience, driving to the clinic late at night, and wandering through the empty corridors to a dimly lit ward, where a nurse gave me the jab. We were able to do it ourselves in later cycles, and most clinics let you do this, but it is vital that you do it at the right time. If there is a problem, and you end up mistakenly doing it later or earlier, you must let the clinic know what has happened. You could put your chances of success at risk if you aren't honest about this.

Immune therapy

This is one of the more controversial areas of fertility testing and treatment, founded on the theory that infertility and miscarriage might be caused by a woman's body rejecting sperm or embryos and preventing a fertilised egg from implanting. Some clinics offer additional tests and treatment to women who've had recurrent miscarriages or repeated IVF failures, based on this idea.

The simplest additional drugs you may be given are aspirin and/or heparin, which are widely prescribed for women who have had recurrent miscarriages. Alternatively, you may be offered other drugs such as steroids or IVIg (intravenous immunoglobulin G treatment), which involves being put on a drip of an infusion of blood products containing antibodies.

Some people swear by these treatments, and believe that they have made all the difference in helping them to get pregnant, but there is no scientific proof for this. The drugs are not licensed for use in reproductive medicine, and there are fears that they could have side effects. They tend to be hugely expensive, and if you opt for the whole range of immune treatments, you could double your IVF treatment bill. Even the doctors who use these drugs admit that there are still many questions about them, and more research needs to be done in this area.

Alison had completed four cycles before she went to a new clinic where it was suggested that taking additional drugs might improve the chances of success:

I felt like I had a sales pitch and had been sold all this extra stuff. There were special drugs to take beforehand and steroids and special drugs to take afterwards. It was just a bombardment of extra drugs and I was so worried about taking steroids. I actually had my worst cycle ever.

Alison's experience is not echoed by everyone who tries these therapies, and many people who have been successful after using them feel they have really made a difference, but you do need to think carefully before going ahead. If you've been through repeated unsuccessful IVF cycles, or have had a number of miscarriages, you may feel that it is worth taking the risk and trying these unproven treatments, but you should discuss it thoroughly with your consultant first. You will need to make sure you are clear about what you are being offered, why the consultant feels it could help in your particular situation, and, most importantly, what the risks and side effects for you and a future baby could be.

Ovarian hyperstimulation syndrome (OHSS)

Hyperstimulation is one of the most serious side effects of IVF, and is thought to occur in around 5 per cent of treatment cycles. Many women have fairly mild hyperstimulation, but OHSS can be extremely serious. It is a direct result of stimulating the ovaries with drugs, and the high levels of hormones in the body are to blame. OHSS does not occur naturally.

If a woman hyperstimulates, her ovaries become enlarged and the balance of fluids in her body is affected. Excess fluid is often found in the abdominal cavity, and it can lead to swelling, dehydration and bloating. Fluid may also collect in the lungs, and if it becomes severe, the condition can lead to an increased risk of blood clots.

Those most likely to develop OHSS are women who have polycystic ovary syndrome (page 10), women who are underweight, those who've hyperstimulated in the past and those who are pregnant with more than one baby. OHSS can develop during the treatment itself, or it can occur as a result of rising levels of hCG in early pregnancy after a successful treatment cycle.

So how would you know if you were in danger of hyperstimulating? Your clinic often has a pretty good idea when they are scanning you, as very large numbers of follicles can suggest that you are at risk, and blood tests will confirm this. You may have discomfort from the enlarged ovaries, followed by swelling in the abdomen, which can cause pain. You may feel nauseous and some women are sick. Other symptoms might include reduced urine output, dehydration and breathlessness.

Toni started to notice that something wasn't right a few days after she'd had her embryo transfer:

> My stomach just started really swelling up, and I started to panic. I rang the hospital and went in for a scan and blood tests. Luckily it was very mild. I only really suffered with swelling and feeling uncomfortable and not being able to sleep. It was really miserable but they don't do anything unless you get it severely.

If ovarian hyperstimulation occurs earlier in the cycle, doctors may want to cancel the treatment immediately, or suggest that you coast for a few days without taking any more drugs, to see what happens. Sarah had symptoms of OHSS before she had her eggs collected:

> They knew there were quite a lot of eggs when they were scanning, but you just swell up because you are retaining tons of fluid. One night I gained five pounds in an hour. I'm usually quite small, and my waist was 34 inches. I did stay overnight in hospital because it is quite dangerous if you suddenly seem to be gaining a lot of weight.

Sarah's condition stabilised and she was allowed to go ahead with her egg collection, but instead of transferring any of the embryos right away, they were all frozen. This is common in such cases, as if you did get pregnant, the pregnancy hormones could aggravate the problem.

Cancelled cycles

When you begin your first IVF cycle, the medical team will be carefully monitoring your response to the drugs as things proceed. We have already seen that if you are at risk of hyperstimulation, it is sometimes necessary to cancel the cycle, and this may also happen if your body is not responding to the drugs. Staff at the clinic may halt the cycle if they don't feel it is worth continuing to egg collection, and they will then modify your drugs regime in the future in order to try to get a better response.

It is difficult if your treatment has to be cancelled, as you will have built up so much hope and expectation, but you should try not to feel despondent. It does happen quite often, and the team will know what to expect next time and will be able to adjust your treatment accordingly. Most clinics offer some kind of refund for cycles that have to be abandoned. The amount you get back is often dependent on how far you have got in the cycle, and you may want to check the clinic policy on this before you start.

Soft, or mild, IVF

Some doctors have become increasingly convinced that it is possible to carry out successful IVF treatment without using as many drugs, or stimulating the ovaries so fiercely. Soft, or mild, IVF has become popular in some clinics. These treatment cycles don't usually start with a period of down-regulation and they use lower doses of stimulating drugs, so women are less likely to suffer adverse reactions or side effects.

Egg collection

When I had my first IVF cycle, I was very excited about egg collection. It had always seemed to be the focal point of the IVF process, but I wasn't at all clear about what was involved and had a hazy notion of some kind of slightly glorified smear test. It was only when the staff emerged in their green operating-theatre outfits that I finally realised the procedure was more of a minor operation than a major smear test. Patients are often asked to get to the clinic fairly early in the morning for egg collection, and both you and your partner will need to be there. You will usually be advised to take the entire day off work.

The semen sample

The male partner will normally be asked to provide a semen sample when you arrive. Men can feel nervous about having to give a sample to order, but by the time you get to this point in the IVF cycle, you are likely to have had some practice at this. Staff are aware that this can be an embarrassing time, and they do try to provide the best environment that they can.

The head of one clinic I spoke to said they had made

an effort to find out what men wanted, and upgraded their 'men's rooms' accordingly:

> It's very difficult to judge what individual patients need and what they want in terms of sperm production. We have very nice rooms with a wash station, a DVD and some magazines, but they don't have to go near any of it if they don't wish to. We also have a range of male vibrators and we can give them non-spermicidal condoms for use before egg collection.

If you have had problems producing a sample to order in the past, alert the medical team to the fact. There's no need to feel any sense of embarrassment. Staff are aware it can be a problem, as this consultant makes clear:

> We use questionnaires with our gentlemen to try and identify whether there is anything we can do to make it easier and more pleasant for them. I think the men are all very nervous. They have to perform under set timing and circumstances away from home, and they're bound to feel uncomfortable and embarrassed.

Although they may feel embarrassed, most men manage to cope with this perfectly well. Najeeb, who has been through four IVF cycles, says some men make too much fuss about it:

> It's the easiest thing in the world to do, and any embarrassment that you might have has got to be seen in the context of what the female partner has to go through. I am

sure it happens; but for me, I didn't feel any pressure or any embarrassment at all.

Sometimes if you are planning to do IVF, and the semen sample is unexpectedly poor, you may be asked for a second sample. The medical team might suggest that you consider ICSI (page 40) rather than IVF if they don't feel the sperm will be able to fertilise an egg without help, and this is sometimes a decision that has to be made on the day.

Preparing for egg collection

The female partner is usually given a gown to put on for the egg collection. You may be wheeled into the operating theatre, or allowed to walk straight in yourself. Egg collection isn't a comfortable process, and you will be given some form of pain relief. Exactly what this constitutes will depend on the clinic. When IVF was first introduced, all egg collections were carried out through a hole in the abdomen, and a general anaesthetic was always necessary. Nowadays, this method is rarely used, and many clinics have dispensed with the need for a general anaesthetic, instead offering some form of sedation and/or local anaesthetic.

Some women say they feel fairly awake during egg collection under sedation, and can recall the process quite clearly, whereas others don't remember anything about it at all. Debbie has had a number of egg collections under sedation, but says she's always felt as if she's had a general anaesthetic:

> The doctors have said I've had mild sedation, but I always
> thought I was knocked out. I've never known a thing about

it. When you see documentaries on television, or when I've talked to other people, they've said it was really painful and they remembered hearing the doctors talking. I never had any of that at all.

After egg collection, I usually had vague disjointed memories of what had happened, and had been aware of some pain when the fluid was sucked from the follicles. I have always been slightly intrigued as to why people have such different reactions to the sedation, and was fascinated to discover from a consultant that this is often directly related to your alcohol tolerance. So, people who rarely drink will be completely out cold after the drugs used for sedation, whereas those who have a fairly high tolerance to alcohol will be far more awake and aware of what is going on.

In theatre

In some clinics, the male partner is allowed into the operating theatre and can stay throughout the process, but this isn't always the case and will depend on how things work at your unit. You may want to ask about this in advance, so that you know what to expect on the day.

Once you are in theatre, the team will usually begin by washing the vagina with cotton wool soaked in saline. Then the egg collection can get underway. It is most often performed by a consultant or doctor, but in some units, nurses are trained to carry out egg collection. An ultrasound probe will be inserted into the vagina so that the follicles around the ovaries can be seen on the screen.

There is a tiny groove down the side of the probe and a thin, hollow needle is inserted into this. The needle is pushed through the vaginal wall to reach the ovaries. Some clinics like to flush out each follicle as they collect the eggs, but others simply suck the fluid out of them. The fluid runs down the needle and into a tube attached to the base. The tube is replaced each time it fills with fluid. The filled tubes are taken straight to the laboratory where an embryologist empties the fluid into a dish and looks at it under a microscope to check for any eggs.

Egg collection doesn't usually take more than half an hour at most from start to finish, and experienced clinic staff can carry out as many as four egg collections in an hour. By the time the procedure is over, the team will have a clear idea of how many eggs have been found in the follicles. An average egg collection will produce between 10 and 12 eggs, but there may be far more, or less, depending on the individual and the level of stimulating drugs used in the cycle. Consultants say that even they can never be sure how many eggs they will retrieve:

We're always trying to do the best for the patient, but you never know what the outcome is going to be. If we know what their anticipation is of the end result, we know whether what has happened in theatre matches that, and can support them through any disappointment they may have. Alternatively, they might think that they were going to get six eggs, and get 16 so they'll be elated.

Patients often feel apprehensive about egg collection, and Lulu admits she went into it full of concerns:

I was very worried that I'd be wide awake and know all about it, and I was anxious because there were all these follicles, but you don't know if there are any eggs in them. Actually I didn't remember a thing about it. I only remember coming round in the recovery room and asking how many eggs I had. It was uncomfortable afterwards, and I was very sore.

I always felt that egg collection was the point I was working towards throughout the treatment cycle, as after that things seem to be taken out of your hands. It seems miraculous, to be harvesting human eggs from your ovaries, but inevitably the process becomes more ordinary when egg collection is part of your normal work routine, as this consultant explains: 'Once you start doing egg collections, and you are doing it regularly, it is like anything else. You do stop thinking about what you are doing. It's very different if you do it as a daily experience.'

It may become familiar, but that doesn't mean the team stop caring about the results. There is a sense of pride in the speed and efficiency with which they can carry out egg collections, and staff admit they find it upsetting on the rare occasions when all the follicles are empty. The focus shifts after egg collection, away from the patient and the medical team, and into the laboratory to the embryologists, who will be responsible for the next stage of the treatment cycle.

Chapter six

In the Laboratory

The next stage of the IVF process takes place in the laboratory. The lab is run by embryologists, and they look after the eggs and sperm, hoping to produce embryos that can then be transferred back into the womb.

A typical day in the laboratory begins early in the morning when the embryologists get into work. In order to make sure that conditions are ideal for any eggs and sperm that arrive in the lab, or for any embryos taken out of the incubators, they begin by carrying out a careful check on all their equipment. It is only once these checks have been carried out, and they are reassured that every-thing is as it should be, that they can get on with the day's work.

Egg collections are often part of the morning's work for the embryologists, but most clinics don't do them seven days a week and the drugs patients are taking are used to help tailor their response so that the eggs will be ready to be harvested at the right time. The medical team are responsible for collecting the eggs, and once this is completed, the embryologists take over for the next part of the treatment cycle.

The eggs arrive in the laboratory

We've already followed your eggs through the door into the laboratory, where the embryologist has tipped the liquid sucked from the follicles into transparent plastic dishes. The embryologist puts the dishes under the microscope and examines them to check whether any eggs are present in the liquid, and if so, how many.

The microscopes used in the laboratory for IVF work are kept behind special glass hoods. This keeps the air circulating and protects the dishes containing the eggs, sperm or embryos from any dust or dirt that could land in them when they are open. The hoods cover only the top of the microscope, so there is plenty of room for the embryologists to work underneath them. The work surfaces are kept warm, so that eggs, sperm and embryos don't get cold when they are being examined.

The recovery room

While the embryologists are starting their work after egg collection, the woman will be taken to the recovery room until she is ready to leave the clinic. Some recovery rooms are like hospital wards with beds, whereas others may be little more than a small room with a chair or two, but you will be able to rest there for a while. The amount of time an individual takes to recover from egg collection depends largely on the kind of anaesthesia the medical team have used. If you have a general anaesthetic, it may take some time for you to come round, and with sedation it is usual to feel woozy for a while. If you are at a clinic that offers a local anaesthetic as an alternative, this can mean a shorter recovery time.

It feels rather odd as a patient at this stage to go home, leaving your eggs and sperm in someone else's hands. It can be reassuring to hand everything over to the experts, but many people are understandably anxious at this point, as everything is out of your control and there is nothing more you can do.

A first look at your eggs

At this stage, the eggs appear under the microscope as round circles. They are surrounded by lots of tiny cells known as cumulus cells, which make it hard to see them clearly. If they are mature, they will have a little bump attached to one side, known as the polar body, and the cumulus cells will be gathered around the outside of the egg like a sunburst. Immature eggs don't have a polar body, as it is not produced until the time ovulation would normally occur. Eggs that don't have a polar body when they are collected can sometimes mature in the laboratory and they may still be able to be fertilised successfully.

The eggs are so tiny that they are invisible to the human eye, and each one will be placed in its own drop of liquid in a plastic dish. The liquid is known as a culture medium, and it has perfectly balanced levels of salts, sugars, protein and nutrients for both the egg and sperm.

If the eggs are going to be used for IVF, there is no need to prepare them first, but for ICSI (page 40) the embryologists have to remove the cumulus cells before they can work with the egg. To do this they suck the egg up in a pipette and then put it into a drop of a special enzyme for up to one minute. The enzyme breaks down the contacts between the cells around the egg so that they come away, and once this has been done, the egg is ready.

Ensuring ideal conditions in the lab

Anyone spending time in a laboratory would be immediately reassured by the level of care that the eggs, sperm and embryos receive. The lab itself is kept warm, and the lights may be dimmed or kept low. At some units, the embryologists even do their own cleaning, rather than risk allowing the hospital cleaners into the lab, to prevent any possible damage to the sensitive eggs, sperm and embryos from cleaning fluids. In other units, the cleaners will be allowed in to mop the floors using special materials that are known to be safe, but a lab assistant may be responsible for cleaning the equipment.

Preparing the sperm

The male partner will have given a semen sample before the egg collection, and the embryologist will have had a look at this under the microscope to get a rough idea of the sperm quantity and quality. The embryologist assesses the sperm in the semen sample, depending on how active and well formed they appear. An embryologist explains:

> We grade them, A, B, C and D. A are the best, very quick and going in a straight line. B are mobile, still moving forwards, but perhaps not so fast, and they may have slightly exaggerated movements. With grade C, there's twitching or

movement on the spot. You can see that they are moving, but they're not going forwards. D are not moving – we use the word 'non-motile'.

The embryologists will not only check sperm quality but also quantity. There are usually millions of sperm in a sample, and you may wonder how on earth the embryologists can count these. They don't sit bleary-eyed counting thousands of individual sperm, but use a counting grid: a slide divided into squares. By looking through the microscope and counting the sperm in just one square, the embryologist can calculate the sperm count by multiplying this by the number of squares.

The semen is prepared before it is used, in order to try to get the best quality sperm from the sample. This form of preparation is known as 'washing'. Washing separates the sperm from the semen, and gets rid of any dead or sluggish sperm as well as any other debris in the sample. The embryologists want to try to harvest all the top-grade sperm from the sample when they wash it, and there are a number of different methods used to do this:

Swim up This process involves putting the semen with a special culture. The sperm try to swim towards it, and the strongest and most active get there first, so these are used in the treatment.

Density gradient sperm wash This process doesn't just sort out the strongest swimmers among the sperm but it will also remove any dead cells or waste products in the sample. Liquids of different densities are put into a test tube with the semen and spun in a centrifuge, which is a bit like a spin dryer. The strongest sperm will make their way to the bottom of the test tube, and any less active or dead sperm will be caught in the upper layers.

Sperm washing Simple sperm washing can be used in conjunction with the other two sperm-sorting techniques, or it may be used alone. The semen sample is put into a test tube with a solution made of protein supplements and antibiotics. The test tube is placed inside the centrifuge and spun around quickly. This spinning process separates the strongest sperm from the seminal fluid.

If the sperm sample is good and there are lots of top-grade sperm, they can be used for IVF. The sperm will be drawn up into a tube, and added to the drops containing the eggs in their dish. The dish will be put into the incubator, where it is hoped that the sperm will fertilise the eggs.

In order to fertilise an egg, one of the sperm has to break through the outer layers that surround the egg, and only the strongest will be able to do this. Once one sperm has got into the egg, enzymes act on the shell to prevent any others breaking through. Usually, the sperm won't manage to fertilise every one of the eggs that have been collected.

ICSI

If the sample doesn't contain sufficient numbers of higher grade sperm to be fairly optimistic about fertilisation using IVF, the embryologists can help by injecting the sperm right into the eggs. This is the process known as ICSI, or intra-cytoplasmic sperm injection. ICSI is carried out using special equipment in the laboratory, sometimes referred to as an ICSI rig or micromanipulator.

Only fully trained and experienced embryologists are allowed to carry out ICSI. It is a delicate procedure, and you can feel assured that they really do know what they are doing by the time they get to this level. Embryologists don't even start ICSI training until they've completed their initial embryology qualification, which will usually have taken at least two years. When clinics are training embryologists for ICSI, they may ask patients if they would be willing to donate any eggs that haven't fertilised, and these will be used for ICSI practice. Once the embryologists have successfully got through this part of the training, they will only be given half the eggs from each egg collection they work on for the first few months, to be absolutely certain that no unnecessary risks are taken.

The workstations used for ICSI look incredibly complicated, and the microscope has an arm on either side. The embryologist looks through the microscope to see the eggs and sperm. The left-hand arm of the microscope has a pipette attached that is used to hold the egg still, and on the right hand is a hollow needle used to suck up the sperm.

The embryologist examines the sperm sample, looking for active sperm that are swimming fairly fast in straight lines. Once a good sperm has been identified, the embryologist uses the needle to break the sperm's tail as they don't want it to be swishing about inside the egg when it is injected in. Then the embryologist sucks up the individual sperm into the needle, tail first so that the head is closest to the bottom of the needle.

The embryologist moves the needle containing the sperm towards the egg, and pushes it into the outer layer until it breaks through. The egg looks a bit like a balloon, as the flexible outer layer bends itself around the needle before it finally bursts through, and the embryologist can squirt the sperm inside.

It is fascinating to watch an embryologist performing ICSI. The care and skill needed to manipulate eggs and sperm that are invisible to the human eye is remarkable, as is the confidence the embryologist has to demonstrate: holding the egg still with the pipette, while chasing the wriggling sperm with the needle and deftly slashing off the tail before sucking it up and injecting it right into the egg.

The incubators

Once the ICSI eggs have been injected with sperm, and the IVF eggs mixed with sperm, they will be left to fertilise. They have to be kept in the correct conditions for this to happen, and the incubators used to store them are maintained at body temperature. The level of carbon dioxide in the air is controlled along with the humidity.

The incubators look like domestic fridges, and are sometimes stacked on top of one another to fit more into the lab. The embryologists keep up-to-date information on the door of each incubator to let them know whose eggs or embryos are inside. This means that they don't have to keep opening the door unnecessarily to find the right dishes.

Inside, the incubators have a second glass door, and then a number of shelves. The eggs will be left in their dishes on the shelf overnight, but there will be a safety system in place to ensure ideal conditions are maintained once everyone has gone home. One embryologist I spoke to described the safety system at her clinic: 'The incubators are all monitored and wired up to a control and alarm system. If they go out of spec during the night, that sets off an alarm system that calls a mobile phone and alerts whoever is on call that night.' The on-call embryologist would be able to check what was wrong immediately and take the necessary steps to sort out any problem, but in reality such alarms are rare.

Have the eggs fertilised?

One of the first jobs for the embryologists when they arrive at work in the morning is to look at the eggs collected the previous day and to see whether they have successfully fertilised. The first signs of fertilisation are two little circles clearly visible inside the egg, which indicate that it has reached what is known as the pronucleate stage.

You will usually get a phone call at some point during the day after your egg collection to tell you whether the eggs have fertilised. It may be the responsibility of the embryologist to make this call, but sometimes a nurse or another member of the team does this. It may not have occurred to you before you start IVF that fertilisation could be a hurdle, and it is often only when you're waiting for this phone call that it strikes you that this is yet another of the milestones on the long pathway through fertility treatment.

If for some reason the eggs haven't fertilised, or you've

only had a low fertilisation rate from a reasonably high number of eggs, you will naturally feel upset. Helena came out of egg collection with 14 eggs, and was anticipating a reasonable number of embryos: 'We left the clinic with such positive feedback: the sperm were good, the eggs were good, everything looked terrific, and then they phoned us the next day and said nothing had fertilised. There was nothing to indicate that might happen, and they said they didn't know why.'

What I hadn't understood until I spent time in embryology labs, was quite how much it affects the embryologists themselves when things don't work out. We tend to see them as professionals who are detached from the emotions we feel as patients. I was amazed when some of them admitted crying after having to ring a patient with bad news, and was impressed by the way they immediately qualified this by saying that however upset they might feel, this was nothing compared to the way the news would affect the patient. One embryologist told me how she felt about calling with bad news:

> It's really upsetting, but you have to remember you're upset because you're giving them bad news and nobody likes doing that, but they're on the receiving end of that news. You have to try to remain professional, because they need you to do your job and to be professional, and to give them all the information that you can.

Not all eggs that fertilise will continue to flourish, and the embryologists wait for the next stage of development when the embryos start dividing before any are transferred to the womb. First, the embryos will separate into two cells, and by the second day they will usually have divided again into four cells. Embryo transfer may take place when they are at the four-cell stage, or the clinic may wait another day and replace the embryos when they have reached six or eight cells on day three. Alternatively, you might wait until they are five days old, when they reach the next stage of development.

Grading embryos

If you have a number of embryos, the embryologists will need to decide which would be the best to transfer. They usually do this by grading the embryos, and it has become common practice in many clinics for the embryologists to tell you the grades of your embryos. The grading systems differ from one clinic to another, and there isn't always consistency across the board about what constitutes a particular grade, or a good embryo.

The grades are based on the appearance of the embryos, and the embryologists will look at how evenly they have divided and whether they can see any bits inside the embryos when they make their assessment. If there are lots of bits inside, the embryo is said to be fragmented. Fragmentation sometimes occurs just after an embryo has divided, and if you look at it again later, the bits may have disappeared. If an embryo has a lot of fragmentation, the embryologists will usually give it a lower grading, as the chances of success are believed to be lower when embryos are very fragmented.

It is important to understand that this grading is based on what the embryologists perceive to be the chances of that embryo implanting successfully, and it has absolutely nothing to do with the health of your future child. This is not always something patients are clear about. When Sarah was told her embryos were not top grade, she was concerned about the consequences:

> We were told that they weren't really the best embryos, but they were pregnancy grade. I thought, *what does that mean? Does that mean the baby will come out with one arm missing?* There's so much that's not explained, and then when you go looking, you're often told that they don't really know.

Sarah went on to have a healthy baby, and the reality is that many people do get pregnant with 'low-grade' embryos, and the grade is irrelevant once an embryo has implanted.

Blastocysts

Some clinics encourage patients who have a number of good embryos to consider leaving them in the laboratory for five days, until they have reached the next level of development. By day four, the embryos have been dividing more rapidly and may contain anything from 10 to 30 cells. Embryos quite often stop growing at this stage, but if they continue developing for another day, they begin to look very different. Instead of an evenly divided cell formation, the embryo will have a fluid cavity containing a lump of cells called the 'inner cell mass', which is the part that will grow into a baby. An embryo that reaches this stage is called a blastocyst.

Pregnancy rates tend to be higher after blastocyst transfer, as the embryos have already gone through a number of crucial stages of development in the laboratory, and putting more than one blastocyst back may carry a high risk of multiple pregnancy.

Patients are often keen on the idea of blastocyst transfer because of the good success rates, but many embryos that start out looking healthy will never manage to develop into blastocysts in the laboratory. Waiting to find out whether they have survived can be hard, as Sandra discovered when she had to make the decision as to whether to leave her embryos the extra few days: 'I must admit it was a tough decision. They said they'd call us if it hadn't got to blastocyst stage and we were getting ready to go to the hospital and dreading a phone call. That was the really tense moment, but we were OK.'

What we still don't know is whether conditions in the laboratory can be as nurturing for embryos as the womb, and whether embryos that don't reach blastocyst stage might have implanted and grown if they were transferred to the woman's body at an earlier stage. Helena's clinic hadn't suggested blastocyst transfer, and it took a bit of persuading on her part to get them to agree to it. Her experiences show how few embryos will get that far in the process: 'We said we wanted to try the blastocyst route. I just felt that from everything I'd read it was more successful. The hospital said if that's what I wanted, they would do it. I had 12 eggs, and nine fertilised, but only two made it to blastocyst.' For Helena, it proved to be the right path, as her treatment was successful, and she went on to have twins.

Witnessing

....

If you spend any time in an embryology lab, you will notice how much time is spent on checks to make absolutely certain that there is no chance of the patients' eggs, sperm or embryos getting muddled up. This is a vital part of what happens in the laboratory, and helps patients to feel confident that their eggs, sperm and embryos are secure.

Every time the embryologists move eggs, sperm or embryos around the lab, you will hear them call for another member of staff to witness what they are doing. The two staff members not only check all the labels on the dishes or straws but also have to record the fact that they've carried out each check as they do it.

Exactly how it is done depends on the clinic, but there is always a labelling system in place with a number of checks to make it very difficult for mistakes to occur. Some clinics use a bar-coding system for their labels, whereas others include a variety of details about the individual patient, such as name, date of birth and clinic number, to ensure there is no room for confusion.

An embryologist explains what is involved in witnessing at her laboratory:

A witness involves two embryologists. Each time you do a witness, you have to sign to say that you've done it. Any time that the eggs and embryos are moved, you both read out the patient's name and date of birth together from the paperwork, and then you'll look at the first dish and read the name and date of birth from there, and then you'll read the name and date of birth from the dish that you are transferring to.

Freezing and thawing

Many people end up with more embryos than they would want to have replaced at once, and will be offered the option of freezing any spare embryos that look good. The idea of freezing life seems extraordinary, and yet it is an everyday part of IVF.

Freezing embryos in the traditional manner takes a couple of hours in the lab. The embryos are dehydrated to reduce their water content, and then frozen in straws. It is important that ice doesn't form in the embryo, and so they are frozen very slowly in what is known as a controlled-rate freezer to stop this happening.

The straws containing the embryos are stored in large tanks of liquid nitrogen at a temperature of -196°C. You may have seen television pictures of these tanks, and the steamy liquid nitrogen that comes pouring out every time they are opened. The straws are clearly marked with all the patient's details, and the embryos can be thawed and used at a later date.

An embryologist described the freezing and thawing process as being a bit like turning a grape into a raisin and then back into a grape again. Unsurprisingly, not all embryos survive this and some will be damaged, so having lots of embryos in the freezer doesn't guarantee that they will all be available for transfer at a later date. Using frozen embryos is a far less invasive and much cheaper procedure for the patient.

Some clinics now use a faster freezing method known as vitrification. Freezing embryos this way takes only about ten minutes and involves using high concentrations of an anti-freeze. The embryos are put into anti-freeze for a short time, and then plunged directly into liquid nitrogen. This method prevents ice crystals forming. Once embryos are frozen, in theory they could be kept indefinitely, but in practice there are legal limits on how long they can be kept in storage and your clinic will be able to explain the rules on this.

The thawing process is fairly similar for embryos frozen using either the slow freezing method or vitrification. Both will be passed through a series of solutions that gradually let the stuff used to freeze them come out of the embryos and allow them to return to normal. For embryos that have been through the slow-freeze method, thawing takes just less than half an hour, but embryos frozen using vitrification can be thawed in anything from 15 minutes.

Preparing for embryo transfer

The embryology team will keep your embryos safe in the laboratory until you are ready to come in for embryo transfer. By this point, you will have had a discussion with them, or a member of the medical team, about how many embryos will be returned to the womb, and about freezing any spare embryos. The embryologists are on hand at embryo transfer, ready with your embryos fresh from the incubator, or ready-thawed if you are having frozen embryo transfer, for the last part of their involvement in your treatment cycle.

Chapter seven

Embryo Transfer

Your embryos will be transferred to the womb between two and five days after egg collection. This will depend on the way things are done at the clinic and the decisions you and the staff have made about what would be best for you. An appointment will be made for you to go into the clinic for the embryo transfer.

How many embryos?

Some people have only one embryo by this stage, which means there is no choice about how many to transfer. For those who have two or more embryos, there may be rules about how many you can put back, which means you won't have a choice in the matter, but you may be asked whether you want to put back one or two embryos. This decision is likely to be dictated by your situation. If you are in your twenties and this is your first IVF attempt, if you've decided to go for blastocyst transfer and have quite a few blastocysts to choose from, then it makes sense to put them back one at a time. If you are in your early forties, have had repeated unsuccessful attempts at IVF, and have two low-grade embryos, you will probably want to put them both back at the same time. In some cases, doctors will transfer three embryos when a woman is in her forties.

When you've been trying to get pregnant for years, the idea of twins, or even triplets, can seem appealing: an instant family in one go, and you may never need to go through treatment again. Some fertility specialists are remarkably laid-back about the prospect of multiple pregnancies, reassuring patients that putting back more than one embryo at a time will increase their chances of success with minimum risk. For some people this may be true, but it really does depend on your individual circumstances.

Fertility specialists don't often spend time on neonatal units watching premature babies struggling to survive, nor do they work with children who have to cope with health problems for the rest of their lives, and this can lead to an assumption that twin pregnancies are just as safe as singleton pregnancies. Although many twin pregnancies will progress without any problems at all, they do carry a number of risks. Twins are six times more likely than single babies to suffer from cerebral palsy and one study found that a third of IVF twins suffered neonatal complications. Twins are often born prematurely, and we know this puts any baby at risk. Women carrying twins are more likely to miscarry, to develop pre-eclampsia (a complication that can occur in pregnancy) or gestational diabetes, and to have problems during delivery.

Sometimes couples going through IVF feel they are happy to take these risks, but it is important to be quite clear that these are risks you are creating, and they are not risks that would exist for your future children if you had one baby at a time. One research project in the UK found that an estimated 220 babies die every year purely as a result of multiple pregnancies after fertility treatment.

Of course, the reality is that most people who are expecting IVF twins will find that they get through the pregnancy without problems. Their babies may be born early, they may spend some time in hospital, but they will be all right. However, a minority will spend the rest of their lives coping with the problems of a multiple birth, and this is not a risk any patient should have to take, or any child should have to live with.

If you do have extra good-quality embryos, you may choose to freeze them and have them transferred later. A frozen embryo cycle is easier than a full IVF cycle, as you will not have to take all the drugs to stimulate your ovaries, or go through egg collection, and it is cheaper, too.

The embryo transfer

You will be given a specific time to get to the clinic for the transfer, which is usually carried out in the same operating theatre as the egg collection. You may be asked to change into a gown for embryo transfer, or to take off the bottom half of your clothes as you would for a scan or a smear test. Most clinics do allow your partner to be present for the embryo transfer, but you may want to check this in advance.

The embryo transfer may be carried out by a doctor or nurse, and it is usually a quick and straightforward procedure. The doctor or nurse will begin by inserting a speculum into the vagina. This is the instrument used when you have a smear test, and it holds the vagina open to give a good view of the cervix.

The medical team may have done a practise embryo transfer at some stage during your treatment, or they may do one now before the real thing, just to make sure they have an idea of the route through your cervix. Usually, doing a mock embryo transfer beforehand will sort out any potential problems, but it is sometimes necessary to use a stiff catheter for transfer, or to hold the cervix open with an instrument called a tenaculum, which can be uncomfortable. In rare cases, it may be necessary to dilate, or open, the cervix in order to put the embryos back, but this would be unusual.

When the medical team are all set, the embryologist will get the embryos ready. This is done at the last minute, so that they spend the minimum amount of time out of the incubator. You may have been given the chance to see your embryos on a screen already, or you may be able to view them now. It can be a strange feeling to see your tiny embryos at this stage.

Sandra has been trying to get pregnant with IVF for some time, and says she always finds it reassuring to see her embryos: 'In most cases, we have been shown the embryos. I found that quite emotional because you are looking at potential babies when you look at them on the screen. I've always found that quite nice, and if it works, you can think that you saw them as embryos.'

The embryos are stored in individual droplets of liquid in their dishes, and the embryologist draws these droplets up into a catheter and then brings them into the theatre. The doctor or nurse inserts the catheter into the vagina and up through the cervix. When it is in the right place, they squirt the embryos out into the womb. They may use ultrasound to see what they are doing, and if this is the case you will probably have been asked to drink lots of water beforehand, as it makes it easier to see what is going on if you have a full bladder. Not all clinics use ultrasound during embryo transfer, as not all doctors believe it is helpful. The embryo transfer is a very quick procedure.

Finally getting to this stage of treatment can feel like a huge achievement, and there is a sense that you are getting close to your goal, as Clare explains:

> I was really excited the first time. They have a slight problem getting my cervix into the right position because I have a retroverted uterus, which is tipped back inside me. The embryo transfer is not very comfortable, but it's not the end of the world, and they showed us on the screen the two little embryos they were going to put back.

Once the contents of the catheter have been squirted out, it is returned to the embryologist who takes it back to the lab to check under the microscope that the embryos have gone. Sometimes they are still in the catheter, and if this happens it will be put back in and the embryos will be squirted out into the womb again.

It's a strange feeling as a patient, knowing that the embryo or embryos that have been so long in the making are now in your body. Women often feel that they should stay as still as possible for as long as possible after embryo transfer, and you will be left to rest for a short while. Most of us feel anxious about having to move about after embryo transfer, and I know I was worried that the embryos were going to fall out as soon as I stood up, but this doesn't happen. There is no evidence that lying down, or sitting still, can have any effect on the outcome; you can be sure doctors would be getting their patients to lie flat for hours if it made a difference to their success rates.

I talked to staff at clinics about this, and although they were aware that patients were often concerned about what they did in the first few hours after embryo transfer, they stressed that there was no need to worry. You are not going to ruin your chances of success if you stop at the supermarket to pick up some shopping on the way back from the clinic, or if you end up having to stand all the way home on the bus.

Sandra has had seven IVF cycles, and says she has become more relaxed about embryo transfer with each one:

> The first couple of times I was too scared to go to the loo, and I was dying to go because you had to have a full bladder for the ultrasound. I was probably over the top, saying, 'Don't drive over any bumps in the car', and I was worried about lifting things. As time goes on, you realise that it doesn't really make any difference. You just have to carry on as normally as you can, but you do tend to want to wrap yourself in cotton wool.

Frozen embryo transfer

If you are having a treatment cycle using frozen embryos, the transfer will happen in exactly the same way. The team will have taken your embryos out of the freezer in advance and left them for a while to make sure that they are still developing. Not all embryos will survive the freezing and thawing process, so having embryos in the freezer doesn't always guarantee that you will have embryos to transfer, but success rates are improving.

Implantation and embryo transfer

Some people assume that having one or two fertilised embryos put into their womb means that they are, initially at least, pregnant. In fact, the crucial factor for pregnancy is implantation, and in order for a treatment to be successful, an embryo has to nestle down into the thick wall of the womb. There is often misunderstanding about this, and an embryologist explained that people do sometimes assume that embryo transfer takes them further down the line towards pregnancy:

> I've had a few people say to me after they've had the embryos put back, 'Does that mean I am pregnant now?' but implantation is the big enigma. In the last 30 years, the way we culture embryos in the lab, the fertilisation rates, and the quality of embryos has all come on in leaps and bounds, but the biggie is implantation. Once you put embryos back in the uterus there are so many factors that can affect it.

The two-week wait

The two weeks between having the embryos transferred and finally getting to do a pregnancy test can seem more like two years. Many women say they find it the hardest part of the treatment cycle, as you are constantly wondering whether it might have worked, and worrying about what you should and shouldn't be doing. I always used to wish I could go to sleep for the whole of the two-week wait, and only wake up again when it was time to do the pregnancy test.

Bed rest

Once you get back home, clinics don't usually advise bed rest, as they don't believe it increases your chances of success. You may find that some books, and some complementary therapists, suggest spending two or three days lying flat, as they claim this can improve your chances of a positive outcome. A number of studies have investigated this theory, and have shown that bed rest after embryo transfer does not improve pregnancy rates. However, if you feel that resting will be calming and relaxing and may help you cope, then you should not feel guilty about doing what is right for you and opting to spend a few days in bed.

I always took the day of the embryo transfer off work and didn't do much, but I couldn't have spent another couple of days in bed. It's a purely personal thing, but it would have made me feel like some kind of invalid. Whatever you choose to do, it may make a difference to how you feel but you can be reassured there is no evidence that it will have any impact on the outcome.

When Kylie went through her first IVF cycle, she was terribly worried about not exerting herself after embryo transfer, but says she's come to realise it doesn't make a difference:

> I think it's one of the worst times. The first time I went a bit over the top and rested a lot and didn't put myself under

any physical stress. I was so worried the embryos were going to drop out. The next time, I tried to keep myself very busy.

Going back to work

If you ask your clinic when you should go back to work after embryo transfer, they will probably tell you that it is entirely up to you, which is not particularly helpful. Some people like to take the entire two-week waiting period off work, because they want to relax and give their embryos the best possible chance of implanting. You shouldn't feel worried or guilty if you want to do this. The two-week wait is an immensely stressful time, and if taking time off work is going to make it easier for you, then you should do it.

A lot may depend on the nature of your job. Some jobs are inherently stressful and demanding, and if you think your work is going to cause problems when you want to feel calm, you might want to consider taking time off, as this fertility nurse suggests:

People say to me, 'Should I take time off work after embryo transfer?' and I say, 'Well, how stressful is your job? If it is going to really get to you, then sign yourself off sick.' In most instances, the job is always going to be there, and surely this is worth investing in just for a short time and then going back.

To tell or not to tell

At this stage in treatment, people sometimes regret having told friends or family the exact timings of their IVF cycle. We were so excited about our first IVF treatment, that we told most of our closest friends and family, and I found it really hard to cope with people who kept asking whether there was 'any news' during the two-week wait, especially as it seemed to start about two days after the embryo transfer. If you tell people, you will have someone to talk to at this difficult time, but you should keep in mind that they may not really understand what you are going through, and you may start to find their interest feels intrusive.

Dealing with your emotions

Emotionally, the two-week wait can be by far the hardest part of an IVF treatment cycle, and it is common to feel very up and down at this stage. Some people find it helps them to think positively about the embryo, or embryos, in the womb, and to visualise them growing and flourishing, but this isn't for everyone. Complementary therapists often suggest this kind of positive thought, and encourage people going through IVF to see themselves with stomachs swelling with pregnancy.

I could never allow myself to believe that the treatment might have worked, because I wanted to protect myself from the terrible disappointment of yet another negative pregnancy test, and was always very downbeat if people asked about it. At the same time, I found myself worrying that my negativity might have an impact on the outcome, and make it less likely to succeed. You can end up going round and round in circles with all this, so try to remember that we all have our own ways of dealing with things, and if thinking one way or another helps you get through it, then that's the best way for you.

Some people find it helps to focus on the positive aspects of the cycle at this stage, and to try to feel reassured that the stimulation has worked, that the eggs have been harvested successfully, that they have fertilised and one or more embryos have been transferred. A first IVF cycle is sometimes a bit of a fact-finding mission, as the medical team are not sure how your body will respond to the drugs, or whether the sperm will fertilise the eggs, and getting as far as the two-week wait is quite an achievement in itself.

Signs of early pregnancy

When you've spent a long time trying to get pregnant, you're likely to be fairly expert on the signs of early pregnancy and it can be tempting to spend much of the two-week wait analysing every tiny physical feeling. Is it your imagination, or do your breasts feel slightly more tender than usual? Do you feel nauseous, or is it just that you've spent the last half hour trying to work out whether you are feeling sick? And does your stomach really look a bit fuller than it did yesterday, or could it perhaps be that you don't usually spend so long inspecting it from every angle in your bedroom mirror?

Clare says she found the two-week wait particularly difficult, and couldn't help constantly wondering whether she was pregnant or not:

> The first week is not too bad because you keep telling yourself it is far too early to feel anything. It is the last few days counting down to the pregnancy test that it becomes really stressful. I would wake up in the morning and wonder

if I felt sick when it was clearly far too early, and you're
running to the loo every two seconds to check whether
your period has started.

Pregnancy advisers suggest that most signs of pregnancy
would not usually appear until after you'd be able to get
a positive pregnancy test result, so even if your treatment
has been successful, you are unlikely to be able to tell
during the two-week wait. Some of the signs of very early
pregnancy can be similar to your usual pre-menstrual
symptoms, and experiencing these doesn't mean your
treatment hasn't worked.

Counselling and support

You may feel that you would like some support from
a counsellor at this point, and if you've turned down
approaches from your clinic about counselling in the
past, that doesn't mean you can't change your mind. You
may find that a local support group, or an online forum,
can be helpful during the two-week wait, as you will be
able to talk to other people who know exactly what it is
like. The online support networks may come into their
own at this stage, and you will find others who are going
through the two-week wait at the same time. This can
be a great time to talk to other people who are feeling
just as obsessed as you are. You can discuss those small,
niggling worries and concerns we all have during the
two-week wait, but would often feel too embarrassed to
bring up at the clinic. Fertility counselling is discussed
in detail in Chapter 9.

What should and shouldn't you do during the two-week wait?

We are all worried about what we should, or rather what we shouldn't, do during this two-week period, and fertility clinics tend to give rather vague advice. More than anything it is a matter of common sense and following your instincts. One fertility nurse I spoke to admitted there wasn't much they could do to help patients at this time. She did say that if you were concerned about anything that might have a negative influence on the outcome of treatment, it was best not to do it:

There is no advice on the whole, but we say if you go to do something and think, *should I be doing this?*, then it's just not worth it during this two weeks. Ladies often ask me about having hot baths, and I can't see any problem with that at all. They should try not to do heavy lifting, but even that probably wouldn't have any effect — it's just for their own peace of mind really.

The clinic will probably tell you not to smoke, and this is one rule you absolutely must follow. We know that smoking has an adverse effect on fertility, and there's really no point in putting yourself through an entire IVF cycle and not making the effort to give up smoking when the evidence is so clear. The same applies to your partner, as smoking can affect male fertility, too, and researchers have found that even passive smoking can make a difference.

You'll probably be told not to drink any alcohol either, and it is worth following this advice during the two-week wait. Although one glass of wine is most unlikely to make any difference to the outcome, you don't want to end up blaming yourself if you've had a drink and then the treatment doesn't work. You should steer clear of recreational drugs, too.

Most clinics also advise couples not to have sexual intercourse during the two-week wait. Again, this is most unlikely to cause any real problems, but if your treatment didn't work, it is something you might blame.

You should have been taking folic acid since the start of your treatment, and you must continue taking it at this time. You can buy it from any chemist or pharmacy. Folic acid is a vitamin found mainly in leafy green vegetables, and helps protect a growing baby from neural tube defects such as spina bifida, which usually occur in the first month of pregnancy. If you've been given progesterone supplements, make sure you use them, too, as there is some evidence that they can make a difference to the outcome of treatment. Women often like to take a multivitamin during IVF to ensure that they aren't missing out on any vital nutrition in their diet, and you can buy special multivitamins for pregnancy and conception that also contain the folic acid you need.

Although a multivitamin may be beneficial at this time, you should aim to get the vitamins and nutrients you need from a healthy diet. You don't need to become obsessive, but you should try to follow healthy-eating guidelines, with a balanced diet of fruit and vegetables, protein, carbohydrate and unsaturated fat. Make sure you are drinking enough water, too. Apart from anything else, you will feel better if you are eating healthily.

If you're having treatment overseas, the chances are that you are going to have to fly during this time, and there is no evidence to suggest that this causes problems.

Some people worry about travelling long distances with newly replaced embryos, but it is not likely to have any impact on the outcome of your treatment, and long flights are only a possible problem much later in pregnancy.

Try to be kind to yourself during the two-week wait. This is a time for going to bed early with a good book, for treating yourself to a haircut or a facial, for taking a long walk, or going for a day out. Life can, and should, go on as normal as far as possible, but it is worth doing anything you can to make it less stressful.

Debbie was told to try indulging herself during the two-week wait, and she says this was good advice: 'It's a joy to think, I've got these two weeks where it is hell and the stress is incredible, so I should just treat myself, watch funny videos and read rubbish magazines and look after myself. Pampering myself has helped me.'

If you are worried about anything during the two-week wait, or if you have any symptoms that you feel are unusual, don't be afraid to contact the clinic. The staff are accustomed to people having concerns at this time, and will do their best to answer your questions. Some clinics do make a point of contacting people at some stage during their two-week wait, just to see how they are getting on, but it is not standard practice, as this nurse explains: 'We advise patients that we won't contact them at all during the next two weeks, but we do remind them of all the telephone numbers, and say that if they have any queries or questions, then they must be in contact with us.'

Sometimes your period will start before the end of the two-week wait, and if this happens you should get in touch with the clinic. They may ask you to do a pregnancy test anyway, as to have some bleeding in early pregnancy is surprisingly common. There is sometimes light bleeding when an embryo implants into the wall of the womb, known as implantation bleeding, or there may be bleeding around the time that a period would have occurred.

Despite all the advice about leading a healthy lifestyle during the two-week wait, there is little that you can do to influence the outcome of your treatment at this stage. Obviously, going on a mad drink-and-drugs binge, or entering a weight-lifting contest, would not be advisable, but people who don't know they are pregnant do all kinds of things they shouldn't in the first few weeks without causing long-term damage to their babies or miscarrying. Perhaps the most important thing you can do is to try to relax, but even as I type the words, I am only too aware what a hard task that can be. It may be more sensible to suggest that if there are things that help you feel calmer and more peaceful, now may be a good time for them!

Chapter eight

The Emotional Impact

When you start IVF, you will probably imagine that getting used to the drugs and the injections, or having to go through egg collection and embryo transfer, will be what makes it difficult. In fact, most people adjust to the physical aspects of treatment remarkably quickly, but find that the emotional side of things is far tougher than they'd anticipated.

The emotional roller coaster

It may have become a cliché, but the experience of going through IVF really does feel like an emotional roller-coaster ride. A treatment cycle consists of a series of hurdles to be got over, and there are so many points at which things can go slightly awry and send you hurtling down to a low, before a glimmer of hope sends you riding up high again. If a scan shows a slow response to the drugs or you don't get as many eggs as you'd hoped for, it may feel like the end of the world, but you may then be ecstatic if you get a good fertilisation rate or top-quality embryos, as Kylie explains: 'You start and you're very excited and full of hope, and then you go on a complete downer and you think it's all lost, and then you're up again, and then down again. The emotional side was hardest.'

These feelings are intensified by the knowledge that so much has been invested in the treatment cycle, both emotionally and financially, and that you are finally close to something you may have been dreaming of for many years. It can be hard to deal with these highs and lows, especially if you are trying to carry on with the rest of your life as normal. Family and friends probably won't understand unless they've had fertility treatment themselves, and you can feel very cut off from those around you.

Isolation and loneliness

You may know that many thousands of other women around the world will be going through IVF at the same time as you, and will be experiencing all the same emotions, but that doesn't stop the feelings of loneliness and isolation that often accompany infertility and treatment. I haven't spoken to anyone who has personal experience of IVF who hasn't felt lonely and cut off from their friends. It is tough when everyone around you seems to be having children without any problem, and when conversation with a group of your peers is no longer about the latest film or favourite restaurants, but suddenly focuses on sleep training and breastfeeding.

Sheila found her sense of isolation grew as she went through fertility tests, and then on to treatment:

When we started trying, just a few of our friends had children, but by the time we were doing the IVF everyone had them, and some people had more than one. It wasn't as bad for my husband, but I felt really excluded because all the other women were talking about things I didn't know about, and going to places you couldn't go without a baby.

Depression

A survey of patients about the emotional impact of infertility carried out a few years ago showed that the vast majority of the respondents had experienced feelings of tearfulness and depression. This isn't always recognised, and couples end up feeling that they are somehow not coping as well as they should if they succumb to depression. Infertility has a deep impact on our general health and well-being, and people who've had their own children easily, or have never wanted children, can't begin to appreciate what it is like to yearn for a child of your own and how this can affect your outlook on life.

Emma says she found going through treatment extremely difficult emotionally: 'I was a bundle of nerves, I was tearful and I found it very hard. It is just a huge burden. It is such a lot to go through emotionally. People have no idea what you are going through and how desperately you want a baby.'

If you feel that you are starting to sink into depression, do something about it. Counselling can be beneficial, and if you don't want to consider that, then make sure you are taking other steps to look after yourself. If things get really bad, don't feel any qualms about going to see your doctor. Many couples going through fertility treatment need emotional as well as medical support, and there is no shame in admitting that.

Loss of control over life

The sense that you have lost control over your life is very common in couples going through IVF. When you first think that you'd like to have a baby, you imagine that you will have some influence over how and when this will happen. The further you get down the path of infertility and treatment, the more this is taken away from you. You find yourself at the mercy of hospital appointment schedules and waiting times for tests and treatments. It can start to feel as if doctors are making all the decisions about what would be best for you, and you are having to fit your life around their schedules.

Unfortunately, the feelings of loss of control often start to spill over into the rest of your life. When you are so focused on getting pregnant and your treatment, you don't have as much time to look after everything else. Your home and work life can seem to spiral away from you, and you may start to feel as if you have no power to alter anything. One woman who was having IVF said it was as if she was 'sitting on the sidelines' of her life, and watching it go by, and it is easy for things to start to feel this way.

Putting your life on hold

It's not easy to carry on leading your life as normal once you are in the throes of infertility and treatment. You're always hoping that you will be expecting a baby by the next month, or the next season, or the next year, and you may not feel able to move house, or apply for a new job, or change your lifestyle. This kind of static life, where everything is on hold, waiting for you to get pregnant, is hard to handle.

Looking back at my career, I had been moving slowly up the ladder until I started trying to get pregnant, and after that I lost all interest in the career path that had seemed so important before we began trying to have a child. There didn't seem to be any point in applying for a new job, as I knew I wouldn't be able to cope with it when I was spending so much time at the clinic and experiencing the emotional upheavals involved in fertility treatment. It's probably an understandable and rational reaction, but if you put too much of your life on hold in this way, it may become a source of resentment and unhappiness if things don't work out to plan.

The constant thought that you 'might be expecting a baby by then' can stop you doing all kinds of things, and it can be difficult to make any plans for the future when you are in limbo waiting for something to happen. The waiting and the uncertainty are part of what make infertility and treatment so very difficult to deal with, as it often drags on far longer than you would ever have anticipated. Some people find it helpful to make a conscious effort not to put things off, but for many others the emotional and financial constraints of treatment make this much more difficult.

Sheila has had three unsuccessful cycles, and admits she feels she can never make any plans for the future:

> We had the opportunity to go skiing last year, but it was going to be just after a cycle and I knew I wouldn't want to go if I was pregnant, so we turned it down. It's stupid because the treatment didn't work, and it would have been really nice to go away, but I do things like that all the time. You're always thinking in your head that maybe you'll be pregnant and you don't like to plan things just in case.

Feelings of shame and failure

You may know perfectly well that it isn't your fault that you can't conceive, but many couples who have fertility problems blame themselves for what is happening, and experience a sense of shame. Having children is something we grow up expecting to be able to do, and when everyone around you seems to be doing it effortlessly, you may feel you are somehow failing.

For men, that sense of failure can be acutely tied in with their male identity and the idea that they must be less of a man if they can't father a child. It's an issue men often find hard to address, and some may not even want to talk about it. It can cause a great deal of guilt when a couple are having fertility treatment for a male factor problem, as it is the woman who has to undergo the invasive treatment. Women can feel resentful about this, although most accept that it is something you are going into as a partnership. Being honest about these feelings and talking them through can help.

For women, the emotional response is similar. We often feel guilty, as if we have failed because a 'proper' woman should surely be able to conceive naturally. Many of us feel that our bodies are letting us down. We may sense that we are inferior to friends who seem to be able to pop out babies easily, and these emotions are deeply set. We know these thoughts are illogical, but that doesn't make them easier to ignore, as Lorraine explains:

> It made me feel like there was something wrong with me, like my body was letting me down. It wasn't doing what it was meant to. I felt as if I was failing my boyfriend, and I was sure it was all my fault that we couldn't have a baby.

Personality changes

Many people say that their entire personality and the way they react to things has altered as a result of their infertility. When you can't have a child, you become more sensitive and touchy about things other people say. You may be overwhelmed with jealousy at the way other people around you seem to have children so easily. People are often shocked by the intensity of these feelings, which may be at odds with the way they see themselves.

Debbie says she found it exceptionally hard to deal with other women's pregnancies when she was trying to conceive: 'It's hard to cope with the jealousy. You feel guilty because you are jealous, and you feel you are a bad person because you aren't happy that someone else has got pregnant naturally. It's perfectly normal, but only people who have been through infertility can understand it.'

It may help if you recognise that it is normal to experience jealousy and anger in the circumstances, but what can be more difficult to deal with is the loss of your sense of fun. It can feel as if infertility is a cloud that has covered your life and is souring everything you do, making it impossible for you to take pleasure from any of the things you usually enjoy.

Relationships

Going through IVF will test your relationship with your partner, but if you are prepared for this and able to talk about it, you may find that will go some way towards helping. Not all relationships will withstand the emotional stresses of infertility and treatment, and about a third of couples feel the experience has a negative effect. It can be particularly difficult if one of you is more dedicated to the process than the other, and this can be a source of great resentment if you haven't talked through your feelings about it at the start.

Conversely, some people find it brings them closer together despite all the stresses and struggles, as Helena discovered when she and her husband went through treatment:

It was amazingly good for our marriage, and I think it bonded us together forever. It has been such a journey – we'd only been married for a couple of years when we started trying and it was a learning experience for both of us. There were times when you felt you were battening down the hatches, and no one else understood.

The sexual side of relationships is often put under a great deal of strain in the lead-up to IVF by the fact that there is no spontaneity when you are trying to time sex to fit in with peak fertility. This is why many doctors recommend that you don't worry too much about this, and instead concentrate on having more sex around the right time. Even that can make sex start to seem like a chore, but once you know you are going to have IVF, you can forget about timings, and one nurse I spoke to says she suggests people use the opportunity to rekindle their relationship:

> We don't tell people to take precautions when they are going through treatment. We say, 'Have lots of sex – we're sorting everything out for you now, so forget all those pressures around "I've got to do it this evening at five o'clock because I am going to ovulate." Wine and flowers; have lots of fun,' and they say it's quite nice because it reinvigorates things.

Dealing with other people

One aspect of living with infertility and treatment that people consistently find awkward is dealing with other people. No one can understand what infertility is like unless they have some personal experience, and other people's impressions of treatment are not always well informed. It may seem as if those around you consistently manage to say the worst possible things when you are feeling vulnerable, but remember that you are likely to be more sensitive than usual and they are not trying to be unkind or hurtful. People will try to give you tips and advice, or helpful suggestions about things that worked for a friend of a friend, and will inevitably tell you about the couple they know who conceived the moment they stopped trying – it's amazing how many people know that couple! It is difficult, but try not to get annoyed, or to let thoughtless comments upset you.

Dealing with family

Your family can be particularly hard work because they will have their own emotional involvement in your fertility problem: your parents may be longing to become grandparents, and your siblings to become aunts and uncles. They want to do what they can to help, but if they try to be too interested, you may feel they are interfering. On the other hand, if they try to avoid the subject entirely because they don't want to upset you, you may start to feel that they don't care.

Isobel admits she didn't find it easy to talk to her family about her experiences of IVF, as the lack of understanding caused real problems:

> There was just a basic communication breakdown. I remember my mum trying to find the right thing to say and coming out with all the platitudes you hear, the things people say just because they don't know what to say, like there's more to life than having children. I said to her, 'You've got three children, how do you know what life without children is like?', and there was tension around that.

How much you tell your family about what is going on with your treatment and when will probably depend on how often you see them, and how close your relationships are. Some people say that their families have given them more support than anyone else, and women who are close to their mothers can find this incredibly helpful when they are going through IVF, but it is by no means a universal experience and for others IVF may put an intolerable strain on family relationships.

Dealing with friends

You are likely to start to feel more and more isolated from your friends if they are all having children at this time. You may find yourself dreading yet another pregnancy announcement, and your social life may also seem to shrink as friends with young children start to lead completely different lives that centre on their families.

Many people say that they lose friends as a direct result of their infertility and treatment. Looking back, I can see that many of my friendships became difficult when I couldn't get pregnant, while friends were on their second and sometimes even third baby. There were certainly some people and certain events that I chose to avoid at times, but this doesn't have to be a permanent change, whatever the outcome of your treatment.

Nigel says that he and his wife lost a number of friends as a direct result of their fertility problems and treatment: 'At one point, we were down to pretty much no friends, and that is very upsetting, as we used to have a large social circle. You start to take it personally and feel isolated, and that people don't care. It weeds out the shallow elements of friendships.'

Part of the reason for these problems with friends is that you are focused on your infertility and treatment, and other people often lose patience. They do not always understand why you are putting yourself through the trials of treatment, especially if it doesn't seem to be working for you. People often assume that IVF will work immediately, and may lose sympathy if it doesn't, as Kylie found:

> A lot of people think if you are going to have IVF, then you are going to have a baby at the end of the year. All our friends turned their backs on us because we had become obsessed with having a baby. They were interested in the first few months, but when it drew out into years, we found that slowly but surely friends began disappearing.

For a single person like Annabel, who is having IVF alone, this loss of friends can be particularly acute: 'I fell out with a lot of my friends when I was going through treatment. All my friends were married or pregnant, or having kids, and I just couldn't be in that environment. I lost contact with a lot of my friends.'

When you can't have another child: emotions and secondary infertility

It is often assumed that couples who are trying unsuccessfully to have a second or third child do not experience the same pain and trauma as those who are trying for a first. To an extent, this may be true, as you won't have that raw fear that you may never become a mother, but you may experience different emotional difficulties. It is more difficult for you to avoid situations where you have to spend time with children, or pregnant women, and you may face endless questions about when or whether you are going to have another child.

Some couples say they find secondary infertility particularly difficult because they want to be able to give their child a sibling, and because they are more aware of the joy they are missing out on. Those around you may not be terribly sympathetic to your situation, and it can be hard to explain the real pain of not being able to conceive in these circumstances. You may feel guilty about accessing the support available to the involuntarily childless when you already have a child, and this can lead to isolation and loneliness.

Your child may have started asking questions about whether he or she will ever have a brother or sister, and it is upsetting when you can't give them an answer. You will have to make a decision about what, if anything, you are going to tell them about your IVF treatment. This may depend in part on their age, as older children will be more aware of visits to the clinic and injections, and are more likely to pick up on what is going on. It can be particularly difficult when you are going through the ups and downs of treatment to try to stay calm for them, and to shield them from your emotions. It is important not to raise their hopes too high about the possibility of having a brother or sister, as this is only going to make it more difficult for you if the treatment doesn't work. If they are old enough to understand, and you want to tell them, it is perhaps best to say that you are having some treatment to try to help you to be able to have a baby rather than being specific about exactly what is going on and when.

What can you do to help yourself?

The experience of not being able to get pregnant and having to go through IVF is never going to be easy or pleasant, but there are ways of making the emotional roller coaster a smoother ride.

Communicate

Perhaps one of the most important ways of getting through this is to make sure you are communicating; making time to sit down with your partner so that you can tell one another how you are feeling, talking to sympathetic friends or family members, and maybe even a counsellor. If you try to keep everything bottled up inside, you're going to feel ready to explode by the end of an IVF cycle.

There's nothing wrong with admitting that you are finding it difficult, and it would be far less normal to find the whole experience a bit of a breeze. IVF can be tough on your relationship, and one way to make sure you and your partner don't let it destroy what you have is to make sure you keep talking to one another.

Information

Once you've stepped onto the conveyor belt that takes you through tests and into IVF, decisions about what you should do and how you should move on may seem to have been taken out of your hands. The best way to take back some control is to make sure that you are as well informed as you possibly can be about the cause of your problem, the treatments doctors are suggesting and the clinics where you might be treated. The more you know, the more you will be able to retain some sense of steering things the way you want them to go.

Sandra says she feels that making the effort to inform yourself can help considerably with this:

> I'm the kind of person that likes to know what is going on, and I would recommend getting as much information as you can. The infertility is out of your control, and I found that reading books and talking about it can help you feel that you are gaining some control back.

It's often hard to concentrate properly during a consultation with a doctor or nurse, and you may find you haven't taken everything in. On the way home from the appointment, you'll suddenly think of half a dozen things you wish you'd asked. If there's something you don't understand, make sure you remember to ask next time you're at the clinic, and don't be worried about sounding stupid by asking them to go over something again. If it's an urgent query, give the clinic a call. Books can be helpful, too, and you may be able to borrow some relevant ones from your local library or even from your clinic or support group.

Most of us turn to the Internet for information now, but do be careful with this. There's a lot of interesting information out there on the Net, but there's a lot of nonsense, too. It can be easy to misinterpret scientific papers that you find online, and sometimes you may read about new theories or treatments that haven't been properly tested, or that have since been disproved. So, although the Internet can be useful, you should be wary of believing everything you read.

Support groups

Joining a support group can be a great help when you're going through IVF. Some clinics run their own groups that may hold occasional meetings, either with guest speakers to address different aspects of fertility and treatment, or just as get-togethers for patients to meet and get to know one another. These kinds of support groups have become less popular in recent years, however, as more and more people look online for support.

There are national support networks in most countries, and these offer a whole range of services, from telephone counselling to information packs on particular problems and treatments. They usually have websites, with forums where you can meet other members and chat, and may run local or regional meetings, and information days. Clare Lewis-Jones of Infertility Network UK says they play an important role in helping people to understand that they are not alone:

> Joining a support network helps remove the feelings of isolation expressed by many of those who contact us. You no longer feel like you are the only person feeling this way or with the difficulties you face. It gives you the opportunity to let off steam and say how you feel – sharing with people who understand, who have 'walked in your shoes'.

You may also find a wide range of support groups for specific fertility problems, and these can be useful whether you need help because you have endometriosis or polycystic ovary syndrome, or are planning to use donor eggs or sperm, or a surrogate. They usually have websites, and are a good source of expert information.

Many also organise meetings and conferences, which can be a great help. There are contact details for many of these organisations in the Resources section at the end of the book.

Internet support

The Internet is not only useful when you are searching for information, but it can also offer support. There are some fantastic online support networks, where you will find posts from people with personal experience of every type of fertility problem and treatment. Many people find online networking extremely helpful, and you may find groups of 'cycle buddies' who are all going through IVF at exactly the same time as you.

The Internet forums have a language of their own, which you will soon pick up once you start reading them. Some sites have useful translation pages to help you make sense of them when you are new. I found it quite hard to fathom some of the postings at first. You may guess that a '2ww' is the two-week wait, and if someone says they have been 'TTC for four years', you may eventually work out that means that they've been trying to conceive for four years, but 'BMS' left me totally confused – that's 'baby-making sex', in case you're wondering.

It is both comforting and reassuring to discover a world where everyone understands how you are feeling, where you can find others at any time of the day or night and get support when you most need it. Some of the online forums organise meetings and events, and people sometimes phone or meet up with friends they've made this way. You've often shared a level of intimacy about your feelings and experiences that you wouldn't normally reveal, and this can create strong and lasting bonds.

Debbie says she's made some good, long-lasting friendships through fertility websites:

> There are girls I've been chatting to on the website for four or five years. We know each other so well, and sometimes we talk every day. I'd love to actually meet them face to face. I met one friend who lived half an hour away and we've supported each other throughout all our cycles. It's a special friendship.

It is sad that these online support networks are almost exclusively the preserve of women. Although there are areas of the sites reserved for men, they are not as busy or as well used. Things are changing slowly, and some pioneering men do post regularly, as they realise that this can be a helpful way of getting support and information.

The one thing you should remember when reading the posts on these forums is that they have been put there by other patients who don't usually have any medical expertise, and the advice they give and suggestions they make are not necessarily things your doctor would endorse. Even the information sections of some of the sites can be inaccurate, so don't believe everything you read unless you've had it backed up elsewhere, as Clare Lewis-Jones of Infertility Network UK warns:

> The potentially bad side of the Internet is that you don't know who you are 'talking' to, or how accurate they are when giving advice. Anyone can set up a website, and some

may demand money and personal identifying details, so couples should be aware of who is behind the websites.

Remember the positive things in your life

You may be struggling to conceive, but try to remember that having a baby is not the only thing that defines us in life. You may have a successful career, a great relationship, a lovely home, good friends and a close family, you may have a talent for art or music, and there may be other things that you've always enjoyed, whether that's travelling, or sport, or gardening. It's easy to forget the good aspects of your life when infertility seems to taint everything, but try not to let it spoil the rest of your life entirely.

When you're focused on trying to get pregnant, it starts to dominate everything in your life, and you may discover, almost without noticing how it has happened, that you aren't making any time to do things you used to enjoy. One fertility nurse I spoke to says she feels people should try to do things that can shift the focus away from IVF and infertility, even if only temporarily:

> I would certainly say to keep a life, keep a grip on reality. We all need a carrot, and every one of us has something different that helps; it might be that you go to the pictures, or you go out for a nice meal with your partner or your friends – or for some people it's the gym.

One of the difficulties many couples face when they are trying not to let IVF dominate their lives, is that the financial burden of paying for treatment can make it very difficult to do the things they used to enjoy. There is not always the spare cash for holidays, or weekends away, or nights out at the theatre, but you don't necessarily need to spend money to have fun, and it may be more a matter of making some time to spend together.

It would be wonderful if you could get so absorbed in other activities that you could forget all about trying to get pregnant, but the reality is that most of us aren't able to do that for more than the shortest interlude. If you can pull your focus away from IVF, it will help remind you that there are still other things in life you can enjoy. It isn't easy, but be kind to yourself, spoil yourself a little, and you will find chinks of light in the gloom.

Chapter nine

Fertility Counselling

Fertility clinics should offer counselling if you are having any kind of assisted conception, but not everyone wants to take this up. If you're the kind of person who has had counselling or therapy in the past, and who knows it has helped, you may be relieved to find a specialist fertility counsellor to help you through treatment. If, on the other hand, you're someone who is deeply cynical about any kind of talking therapy, then you may feel any suggestion that you should see a counsellor is intrusive. In the middle are those who don't have any strong feelings about counselling either way, but who may worry that rushing straight off to see the counsellor would mean admitting that they were not able to cope.

Most professionals in the field suggest that patients at least consider counselling. They know how difficult an IVF cycle can be, and how much some people struggle. They have also seen at first hand how supportive counselling can be.

Types of counselling

There are a number of different types of counselling that you could be offered, depending on your individual needs and circumstances.

Support counselling

Most of the counselling that takes place in fertility clinics is support counselling. This type of counselling focuses directly on how you are coping with your infertility. In a support counselling session you will talk through your feelings, and the counsellor will aim to help you to try to work out some strategies for dealing with them, and for making the experience of going through treatment more bearable.

Implications counselling

This is used when patients need to think through the implications of a specific type of treatment, perhaps when they are going to use donated sperm, eggs or embryos, or are planning a surrogate pregnancy. Implications counselling aims to ensure that you have thought through the implications of the treatment you are about to undergo for everyone concerned.

Therapeutic counselling

Most counsellors working in fertility clinics don't get involved in much therapeutic counselling. It would take in other issues in your life, and might look at the underlying reasons why you want children. It could be used if there are problematic issues in your past, or if you are having difficulties in your relationship. It is very time-consuming, and the more immediate assistance offered through support and implications counselling will be more relevant for the majority of those in the fertility clinic.

Finding a counsellor

Fertility clinics may have an in-house counsellor or you may be given contact details of someone you can go to see at their own practice. All clinics should have links with a counsellor, and should be able to recommend someone who has experience at dealing with fertility patients.

If a counsellor has been recommended by the clinic, they should be qualified and accredited by the relevant governing bodies. If for some reason you are not happy with the counsellor the clinic recommends, or if you want to find an independent counsellor yourself, you should check that he or she has counselling qualifications and is a member of a professional organisation.

Some patients opt to see a general counsellor, which can sometimes be arranged through your doctor, and find that this is helpful. It is generally worth trying to find a counsellor who specialises in infertility, if you can. They will be more aware of the specific problems and emotional difficulties you are facing, and will have more experience of finding the right kind of coping strategies to deal with them.

I went to see a general counsellor when we were still waiting to start IVF, and it convinced me of the need to see someone who has experience of dealing with infertility. The counsellor was more interested in the aspects of my family history that might have led me to want children of my own, than in my inability to conceive. While I have no doubt that there are deep-seated links between our backgrounds and our desire to conceive, they didn't feel important to me at that time when I desperately needed some kind of support to help me cope. My doctor had suggested that a counsellor could give me some strategies for this, but instead I emerged from the session feeling worse than I had when I went in. If you see a counsellor who specialises in infertility, you are far more likely to find it beneficial.

What happens in a counselling session?

Most counsellors like to try to see both partners together for the first session if they are having treatment as a couple. The counsellor may have had a look at your medical notes before the session begins but this is not always the case, and they will sometimes ask you to start by explaining your individual situation.

Counselling is often a tearful process, and counsellors always seem to have a box of tissues ready for this eventuality. You should never feel embarrassed about crying during the sessions, as you are likely to be addressing some difficult issues. Facing up to your problems and trying to deal with them is a sign of your emotional strength rather than weakness, but it can be an upsetting process.

Exactly what goes on during the session depends on the individual and the counsellor, but in support counselling you will often try to work together to find ways to make your situation easier, as this counsellor explains:

What we would hope to do is initiate some coping strategies which may perhaps just include taking time out, and taking time to relax. Going through such treatment is a punishing regime for anybody, and I think if people were suitably prepared emotionally, then physically they would cope with things so much better.

Coping methods vary from person to person but they may involve finding time for yourself to do things you enjoy, either individually or as a couple. One counsellor I spoke to said she hoped patients would feel that they had left some of their sadness and stress behind after a counselling session, which is a lovely idea. It probably works to a greater or lesser degree depending on the relationship between the individual and the counsellor. You may find that the first counsellor you see just isn't right for you, and that you don't feel comfortable with the sessions. This doesn't necessarily mean that counselling is not for you, as sometimes in such circumstances people find they can get more out of the experience if they seek out an alternative counsellor.

Someone to talk to

People can be put off counselling because they fear that they will be forced to open up about emotions that they may be carefully keeping under wraps in order to cope. In fact, it is up to you what you choose to disclose during a treatment session, although you will get more out of it if you are able to be honest.

A counsellor can just act as a sounding board: someone to talk to who doesn't have any emotional involvement in your situation. People often worry that they are starting to bore their friends or family, who can't fully understand what they are going through, and a counsellor won't be making value judgements or allowing their own feelings to influence the situation.

Counselling may also help you identify some of the areas of your life that are particularly stressful as you go through treatment, and then to work out how to eliminate some of the stresses that may exacerbate a fertility problem, as this counsellor explains:

> When we are stressed, our whole body tends to invest energy in coping with the stress, and less energy in coping with the problem. I have no doubt that stress perpetuates infertility, but there are all sorts of other contributing factors. We try to look at ways to minimise some of the stress factors that are contributing to infertility.

Lulu only ever had one counselling session during her IVF treatment, but she says she found it a positive experience: 'I had a session after the embryo transfer. It was really just to pour out my anxiety. I think it was useful just to have a place to offload yourself to somebody.' Lulu's experience illustrates that just one session at the right time can make all the difference, and if you feel at any point during your treatment that you need someone to talk to, don't forget the counsellor.

Privacy and counselling

Many of the patients I've spoken to have expressed concerns about how much of what goes on in a counselling session gets back to the rest of the team treating them. People are sometimes worried about discussing any doubts or negative feelings they may have, in case this somehow prejudices their treatment. It is often particularly acute for those who are going to be using donor eggs, sperm or embryos and who may feel that the counselling session is some kind of test, with right and wrong answers.

All the professionals working in clinics that I interviewed were keen to explain that they had no idea of what goes on during the counselling sessions. If a counsellor is particularly concerned about someone they are seeing, they don't go straight back to the other staff and tell everyone. Instead, they would first discuss their concerns with the patient, and would come to a mutual agreement about what would be said to the rest of the team. For the most part, doctors are aware that their patients are using the counselling service only if they choose to tell them, as this consultant makes clear: 'Counselling is completely independent, and none of it comes back to us. The patients book their appointments with the counsellor independently and we don't know who is going to see the counsellor or what they discuss.'

Getting support at the start

One of the problems with counselling is that it may not always be offered at the time when you most need it. There may be a crunch point when you first get the diagnosis that you have a fertility problem, or are told that you may need treatment if you are ever going to have a child of your own. One fertility nurse I interviewed felt very strongly about this:

I wish there was more counselling available to couples at the point when the bad news first starts to come in. It wouldn't suit everybody, but I think if people had support right at the beginning, it would make having treatment so much better and would give them the inner strength to make the decisions about how much treatment they are going to do.

Her views were backed up by one of the consultants, who thought that people should always consider counselling early on:

There are some couples that cope with it all very well, and others that are not able to cope at all. I always suggest that if you think you are not going to be able to cope with it, try and see a counsellor before you start the treatment, not when your treatment has failed. It does help. ——

Crisis points in treatment

It seems that the majority of patients decide they don't want counselling, and sometimes this is because they turned it down at the beginning, and may have felt it was too late to change their minds when problems arose. Clinic staff say people rarely appreciate how difficult IVF might be when they start out, as this nurse explains:

When you start having treatment you are optimistic. You know the chances of success, and there is a tendency to think, *well, I won't be part of the 60 or 70 per cent that aren't going to be successful.* After that first treatment cycle, I think people can have quite a significant plummet emotionally.

Doctors and nurses usually tell their patients about the counselling services when they are about to start treatment, and if you are adamant at this stage that you don't want counselling, they may not mention it again when there are so many other things to discuss in appointments further down the line. You should be able to access the counselling service when you need it, and opting to see a counsellor in the middle of a cycle if you're finding it tough is perfectly acceptable. The only problem with doing this is that you may not be able to get an appointment right away, but this will depend on how busy the counsellor is. If you feel it is urgent, they may be able to refer you to someone else.

Sarah didn't have any counselling when she went through IVF, but in retrospect she feels it would have helped:

> You have no idea what it is going to be like until you are in the middle of it, and then you are a complete hormonal mess as well. It was awful. I remember at one point the clinic saying, maybe you should speak to our counsellor, and I said OK, but it was two months before she even had an opening.

Post-treatment counselling

Most clinics will offer you an appointment at some point after an unsuccessful cycle to discuss what might have gone wrong, and to make a plan for the future. Sometimes, patients don't want to take this up, perhaps because they've decided they don't want to have any more treatment, can't afford any more treatment, or want to try another clinic. People are not generally offered counselling at this stage, although it could be particularly helpful.

Kylie has been through a number of IVF cycles, and she feels counselling should be offered all the way through. She believes the only way to ensure everyone reaps the benefits of counselling is to make it mandatory:

> If it was part of the treatment, so that you had to do it, then people would accept it. If it is optional and people can avoid it, then they just think it is annoying. I feel anybody going through fertility treatment must do this first. It would save so much heartache.

Men and counselling

Men tend to be particularly resistant to counselling, and although they may agree to come along to a counselling session with their partner, it is often the woman who will make follow-up appointments and come to them alone. One counsellor I spoke to said she had noticed that men tend to shut off problems, believing that if you can't solve something you wrap it up like a parcel and forget about it. She said that although some women may do this too, they tend to keep taking the parcel out to have a look at it!

Counselling for donor gametes and surrogacy

Your clinic may insist that you have a session of implications counselling if you are going to be using donor sperm, eggs or embryos, or if are considering surrogacy. This will also apply to anyone who is thinking of donating eggs, sperm or embryos, becoming a surrogate or joining an egg-sharing scheme.

Most people recognise that clinics need to feel confident that they understand the implications of some of these more complex arrangements, and are happy to attend the counselling session. Indeed, some feel that one single session with a counsellor is simply not enough to get through all the complex issues involved, but a significant minority are less happy about it, and see mandatory counselling as an invasion of their privacy. Whatever you feel about it beforehand, staff report that patients are often surprised by how helpful this counselling can be, as a fertility nurse explains: 'I've found that patients who arc quite verbose about not wanting to go will quite often say afterwards that it was a real eye-opener, and raised things they had never even considered.' You will find more information about counselling for donor treatment in Chapter 11.

Counselling is not for me

Some people don't want or need counselling. You may feel you can talk to your friends about the issues you want to discuss, and that you have adequate support from those around you. Friends, family, complementary therapists and even the other staff at the clinic may be there to listen when you need someone to talk to. You may want to consider whether there would be an advantage to talking to someone who can devote time to listening, but you might still conclude that counselling isn't for you.

The counsellors I spoke to were aware that some people were deeply sceptical about counselling, and one admitted that this can make their job more difficult:

> There are an awful lot of people who are very cynical about counselling and therapy, and with that cynicism they are not going to benefit. What they are cynical about could be a whole area for exploration, but it's not our job to get them over that. People only benefit if they are receptive, and those who come in guarded and defensive will not benefit in any way.

Whatever your thoughts on counselling, you should keep in mind that if at any point before, during or after your treatment you are finding it hard to cope, you have nothing to lose by making an appointment to see a fertility counsellor. It may not help, but when you are going through something as difficult as IVF, it is worth trying something that so many people have found beneficial. You never know, you may be pleasantly surprised.

Chapter ten

The Male Perspective

When I started looking for interviewees for this book, I was overwhelmed by the response from women who were willing to bare their souls and discuss their feelings about infertility and IVF. When I tried to find some men to talk to for this chapter on the male perspective, there was a deafening silence. Eventually, I did manage to track down a handful of men who agreed to talk to me, but it had taken far more time and effort than it had to find their female counterparts.

The reluctance to talk to strangers about such deeply personal matters is understandable, but men's unwillingness to talk even to one another is reflected on the Internet forums dealing with infertility. They are jampacked with women discussing the most intimate details of their problems and treatment in public with people they've never met, but postings by men are relatively rare.

When Dave found out he had a fertility problem, he thought the Internet would be the ideal way to get in touch with other men, as his partner had been happily chatting away to other women on fertility websites:

'There was a room they'd set up for men on there. I put a post on saying, Hi, I'm Dave, I've got this and this, and my wife's got this and this. It was four months before another bloke replied.'

Dave's experience doesn't surprise those working in the field. Women are far more active when it comes to seeking support, as Clare Lewis-Jones of Infertility Network UK explains:

> There are more men getting in touch than 10 or 15 years ago, but they are still in the minority. We have a forum on our website for 'men only', but very few use it. It's a shame because men would, and obviously do, benefit from being part of a support network. They find it perhaps more difficult than women to ask for support and/or talk about their feelings.

Male fertility problems: diagnosis

It is true that for some men, the diagnosis of a fertility problem can strike to the heart of the way they feel about themselves. There is an idea that having a low sperm count makes you less of a man, that the ability to procreate is linked to a man's masculinity, and that men who have lots of children are particularly macho. It is also sometimes assumed that men who appear to be very masculine, muscular and hairy must have a higher sperm count than their small, slim peers.

In fact, all of these assumptions are completely false. A man's sperm count has nothing to do with his physical characteristics, which are largely inherited. Nor does the sperm count bear any relation to his sex drive, which is regulated by levels of testosterone. Testosterone is the hormone that makes men have deep voices and grow beards and body hair, but it is not the main driver when it comes to sperm production. High testosterone levels don't lead to a high sperm count.

Even when you are aware of all this, it can still feel pretty grim when you are given the results of a semen analysis that show a low sperm count. Dave admits that getting his results left him feeling distraught:

> The semen analysis showed I had a count of less than one million, and they did another test on the sperm efficiency that wasn't even high enough to count. It was quite devastating. It felt like you weren't really a man, and having grown up expecting certain things, it was all taken away.

You should be aware that sperm counts can vary considerably, and may be affected by a bout of heavy drinking or illness. If you get a result that causes concern, it is worth having it repeated to be sure it is giving an accurate picture. Fertility clinics often like to do their own tests, even if you've had a number done before at your doctor's surgery or local hospital, and you may be asked for more than one sample to confirm a result.

Sometimes, a closer and more detailed analysis can find a problem that wasn't discovered initially, as Nigel learned when he went for a test:

> I'd always felt, although I didn't have anything to base it on, that there was a problem, and I expected to get a bad result. I did my test at my clinic and when I was told everything

was fine there was just massive relief. Then my wife took my results to her clinic and they looked at them and said there was a serious problem. I went for another test, and there was clearly an issue.

Treatments for male infertility

The type of treatment offered for male infertility will depend on the cause and nature of the problem. Drug therapies or surgery can sometimes help, and intra-uterine insemination (IUI) may be suggested for mild male factor problems. If there is a minor problem with the sperm, IVF can sometimes be used successfully, but the embryologists will want to be certain that the sperm count is going to be high enough for the sperm to fertilise the egg without any help. In a borderline case, they may decide on the day of collection whether the sperm sample looks as if it will be suitable for IVF. If there are concerns, the embryologists are likely to play it safe and opt for ICSI (page 40), as this will give a better chance of success when the sperm count is low. If there are more serious male factor problems, it may be necessary to retrieve sperm surgically, and then to carry out ICSI.

Vasectomy reversal

Men who have chosen to have a vasectomy either because they didn't want children, or didn't want any more children, sometimes come to regret their decision in later years. It is perhaps most common for men who have been sterilised to change their minds when they enter into a new relationship, and decide that they would like children with a new partner.

Vasectomy involves cutting or blocking the tubes that carry the semen from the testicles down into the penis. Attempting to reverse this and repair tubes that have been cut or blocked is a delicate operation, and it is not always a success. The likelihood of the reversal operation working is linked to the amount of time that has passed since the original vasectomy, and if it is less than five years there is more room for optimism. Generally, it is estimated that around half of vasectomy reversals are successful, and this highlights the fact that vasectomy is not a method of contraception to be chosen lightly. If a vasectomy reversal doesn't work, a pregnancy may sometimes still be possible by surgical sperm retrieval with ICSI, but success is far from guaranteed.

Using donor sperm

As we've seen, the latest techniques in reproductive technology have allowed many men to father their own biological children when this wouldn't have been possible just a few decades ago. Despite all these advances, there are cases where doctors cannot get around the problems, for example where a man is not producing any sperm at all, and then donor sperm may be the best way ahead.

Some men come to terms with the idea of donor sperm fairly quickly, but for others it can be more difficult. You will want to make sure you have understood all the implications, and you may find it helpful to talk to others who have used donor sperm about their experiences. There's more information about this in Chapter 11 on using donor sperm and eggs, and there are details of organisations that can help in the Resources section at the back of the book.

An IVF/ICSI cycle

Once you've decided to go for a cycle of IVF or ICSI treatment, the attention will focus on your female partner. She's the one who will be taking the drugs to stimulate her ovaries, going through the egg collection and having the embryos transferred to her womb, even if she doesn't have any kind of fertility problem herself.

Men can feel guilty about this, and sidelined by the fact that the woman has to take on the bulk of what is involved in treatment. You should not underestimate how important your role can be in terms of support, or how much difference this can make. Jo was aware that her partner felt bad about her having to go through so much at this stage:

> I know he felt guilty that it was me who had to have all the treatment when it was his problem. I didn't see it that way, though. I didn't want to go off with the first guy who came along with a high sperm count. I didn't want just any baby, I wanted our baby, and this was what we had to do.

Preparing for treatment

Before you start treatment, we know that women should be in the best possible health, but this is equally important for the male partner. If you are smoking, drinking too much and eating unhealthily, it will affect the quality and quantity of your sperm. The sperm production line

takes nearly three months from start to finish, so you
should try to keep as healthy as you can in the weeks
leading up to treatment.

When Emma and her partner went through treatment,
they were both very careful about what they ate and
drank, and they found it paid off:

> He cut back on alcohol totally, just having the odd glass of
> wine now and again. We were really good with our fruit
> and veg, and he took multivitamins and zinc supplements.
> It really made a difference when we were having his sperm
> checked – the volume and everything had increased.

There are some environmental factors that are thought
to contribute to male fertility problems, and if you regularly come into close contact with pesticides or other
chemicals, you should discuss this with your doctor.
Sperm counts can also be affected if the testicles are
exposed to excess heat, and that is why you may be
told to avoid spending too long in the sauna or hot tub
at this time. This is also behind the advice that men
shouldn't wear restrictive, tight underwear if they are
trying for a baby.

Going to the clinic

Once you get into the swing of treatment, many of the
appointments can be attended by the female partner alone,
and women often go by themselves for most of the scans
and blood tests. At this stage, women are more involved in
the process. Most of it happens to them physically, and this
can lead to them being more emotionally involved, too.

Not all couples want to attend every appointment

together, but some believe it is important to support one another, as this is, after all, a joint project. Nigel always went to the clinic with his wife throughout all their fertility treatment, and soon became aware that many male partners didn't turn up:

> I did notice lots of women by themselves in clinics, and I was quite surprised by that because I can't imagine a scenario where you'd let your partner go without being there. I just can't understand that. It's a tough thing to go through, and you need to support each other.

Najeeb felt the same way:

> I wanted my partner to feel like I was involved because it is really hard on women. The male role in the whole cycle of IVF is almost 100 per cent emotional support, and all the physical symptoms and treatments, and all the discomfort, is down to women. If my partner went for a blood test, I went with her, if she went for a consultation, I went with her. I felt it was important that she had that support.

Some men say they feel uncomfortable at the clinic, but this is not a male preserve. Many women feel just as uncomfortable, but they don't have any choice about whether they attend or not. Clinics don't always help men to be as involved as they could, and this may affect the way they feel about going to appointments, as Graham found when he took time off work to go with his partner:

> It was quite hard for me to get the time off work, but every time I went, I ended up wondering why I'd gone to all the

trouble of getting someone to cover for me. I didn't feel involved at all, and I just kind of sat there and watched.

It is a good idea to discuss how you both feel about this before you start treatment. It may be that it is simply not viable, either financially or logistically, for both of you to take time off to go to the clinic when the male role will be largely a supporting one. You might feel that it is a waste of time for you both to go to every appointment, and some women may actually prefer to go alone. It is true that more men are attending appointments with their partners now, and feel that it helps reinforce the fact that this is something they have gone into as a partnership. It isn't for everyone, though, and you should do whatever suits you both best.

IVF injections

Practically, one thing many men can do to get more involved is administering the injections for their partners during IVF. It can help a man to feel less of a bystander in the process if he can do the injections, as Graham found: 'I was worried about having to do it. I don't like needles, and I'd expected it to be scary. In fact, once I'd done the first one, it really wasn't that bad at all. I think I got quite good at it in the end.'

Najeeb did the injections for his partner, too, and he believes men should all be able to help this way:

I actively asked to do it, and I think it's something they could promote more. Any man is able to administer an injection if he's given ten minutes' guidance on how to do it. It helps them become involved, and it helps the female partner to think he's doing something. It is inflicting pain, but as a man it is good to see that the injections are hurting, because it gives you an appreciation of what they're going through.

Supporting your partner

However involved you may want to be in the IVF process, the reality is that most of it will be happening to your partner. Despite this, your role offering emotional support makes all the difference to how she manages to cope with it.

You should appreciate that the drugs used in IVF can have side effects, and if your partner begins the cycle by taking down-regulating drugs (page 78), these send her body into a premature menopause, which can have some unpleasant reactions. She may have hot flushes, night sweats or headaches, and feel depressed or experience mood swings. These hormonal reactions will come on top of the emotional stresses of the treatment itself, and it can be very difficult, in fact pretty much impossible, to remain calm and relaxed throughout.

Supporting your partner through this can be difficult, and you are going to have your own emotional responses to deal with, too. Nigel feels men aren't always aware of what they're taking on when they start IVF, and that this can make it more difficult:

A lot of guys enter IVF thinking, *test-tube baby, we'll nip up to the clinic and it's a quick process.* It's very emotionally draining and all-consuming, and the most important thing is to make sure you want this as much as your partner, because if you don't, you'll resent them all the way through.

Women can be more motivated than their partners to start on the path towards tests and treatment for a fertility problem, and the biological clock may be partly responsible for this. Knowing that you can probably still father a child way past middle age allows men to adopt a more relaxed attitude. Staff at fertility clinics are sometimes aware that a couple are not entirely united in their desire for a child, and a fertility nurse I spoke to said that men often find it hard to admit they find IVF difficult to cope with: 'Men struggle so much, and not many men can say, "I am finding this hard and I don't like it." Generally, they are coming to the unit because it is the woman who has pushed, although there are some men who are more desperate than their partners.'

Going through treatment together is a real test of a relationship. You may have already experienced difficulties during the time you have spent trying to have a child, when sexual relationships suffer as you try to time intercourse to fit with the most fertile periods during the month. It can take a while for the spontaneity to return, but once you start down the path to IVF, you can try to reinvigorate that side of your relationship, as you no longer have to worry about timing.

Dealing with your own emotions

There is a danger that you can become so focused on supporting your partner and trying to remain in control that you don't always get the help you need yourself. Men often feel guilty about their infertility, and, as Dave explains, may worry about letting their families and partners down:

> It's a natural instinct to want to reproduce, but once you get told that you can't, the feelings grow more and more. It's the only thing in the world you want. I can't give my parents grandchildren, and I can't give my partner children. I feel guilty sometimes and it worries me that at some point in life, my partner will think, *I want children more than I want to be with Dave*, and leave.

It can be hard for men to admit that there is an element of fear and insecurity involved, and keeping this bottled up inside is tough, as Clare Lewis-Jones of Infertility Network UK explains: 'I think many men feel they have to be the strong one emotionally, to support their partner. I also think that, sadly, they are worried that their male friends and colleagues will not understand, they see it as an attack on their virility and fear inappropriate remarks.'

Dealing with other people

Other people are going to say the wrong thing, and this is something you just have to accept. Often friends or family are trying to be helpful, but don't really know how to deal with infertility. In an all-male environment, there can be a tendency to joke about fertility problems, and men may find themselves becoming the brunt of what friends may feel are light-hearted comments; for example, being teased about 'shooting blanks' or being a 'Jaffa'. Friends may not realise how hurtful this kind of remark can be, and are not necessarily trying to be malicious, but may feel embarrassed themselves, and uncertain how to deal with the situation.

The other thing you may encounter is an assumption that male infertility is linked to impotence, and that you have a sexual problem. This kind of ignorance is becoming less common as people are more open about infertility, but there is still a lot of misunderstanding. Nigel feels men just have to learn to cope with all this:

Anybody going through this will have their relationships with friends and family tested. You have to deal with insensitivity, and you have to develop a bit of a thick skin and remember that their intentions are fine and they are trying to say the right thing, but just don't know what to say.

Support groups

We've already established that men tend not to be as keen as women to discuss their fertility problems online, and the same goes for support groups, too. If your local hospital runs a support group, or there's a local network group, this can be a good way of meeting other men, as couples often go together, and it will give you an opportunity to discuss things you may not normally feel able to talk about.

When we first went to a patient support group meeting, we nearly didn't make it through the door. We spent the journey there wondering why on earth we were driving for 40 minutes to spend an evening with people we'd never met, and kept reminding each other that we weren't the kind of people who went to support groups. I'm not entirely sure what kind of people we imagined did go to them, but I suspect every single person who went to the meeting had exactly the same doubts about it beforehand. We were surprised that we both found it a helpful experience, and some of the men in the group were able to be very vocal about their feelings and experiences. If you do have the opportunity of joining a local group, give it a try. If you don't like it, you don't have to go again.

Men and counselling

Counsellors report that men tend to be less enthusiastic about coming along to their sessions, too. Men often go along to the first appointment with their partner, but rarely choose to make their own appointments to see the counsellor. A counsellor at a clinic that carries out about four hundred treatment cycles a year told me that fewer than a dozen of the men going through IVF in that period would see her on an individual basis.

Counselling is not for everyone, but there's little to be lost by trying one session, and you may, like Najeeb, find it does have some value. He went for an appointment with his partner before they started treatment:

> Before our first cycle we had counselling and that was really useful. We haven't had any further counselling since, but we haven't felt we've needed it, I think counselling is useful.

The counsellors I've come across want to talk about how it would affect your relationship and that kind of thing, so it's useful from that point of view.

It isn't always easy to admit that you are finding it hard, but men are increasingly aware of the benefits of seeking support. If you can do this, it may make all the difference, not just to how you and your partner cope with IVF, but also to your relationship in the future.

Chapter eleven

Using Donor Sperm and Eggs

If you are using donor sperm, eggs or embryos for your IVF treatment, there will be some additional practical and emotional issues to address. There are often far longer waiting lists for treatment, it will cost more, and you need to have thought through the long-term implications for not just yourself and your partner, but also your future children.

Donor sperm

Men with fertility problems have made use of donor sperm for decades, and you can either do this during a simple intrauterine insemination (IUI) cycle, or with IVF if there are also female fertility problems. Lesbian couples and single women can use donor sperm in the same way, either with IUI or IVF.

There is an international trade in sperm, with countries that have severe shortages importing semen samples from other countries where there are well-stocked sperm banks. There may be strict regulations for importing sperm between countries, and this can make it difficult for those who want to use sperm from overseas because of shortages at home. Countries which have ruled that all donors must be identifiable will often not allow imports of sperm that was donated anonymously.

No one feels instantly happy about using donor sperm, and it will take time to think through all the implications for the future. Nigel and his partner had originally been told that they could use Nigel's own sperm with a donor egg, and he had some worries about this: 'I was quite pleased that the child would be genetically mine, but very conscious that it wouldn't be genetically my wife's. I did have a bit of an issue with it and was very concerned that it wasn't fair.'

Eventually, they had to use both the egg and sperm from donors, and Nigel says he found it surprisingly easy to come to terms with this, particularly as it addressed his earlier concerns: 'I had a bit of internal sadness, but it was outweighed by the positives. Our desire to be parents outweighed the fact that our children wouldn't be genetically ours, and the option of using donor sperm balanced the equation.'

Reputable clinics have strict regulations about sperm donors, and will check them thoroughly before they are able to make donations. Their samples will have been frozen to give the clinic time for thorough and repeated testing for sexually transmitted infections and a range of inherited conditions, so that you can be sure the sample you get is as safe as possible. There will be an attempt to match the donor to your requirements, although how close a match you get may depend on the number of donors available.

Sometimes lesbian couples or single women may wish to use a known donor: a friend who has decided they would like to donate. Some heterosexual couples choose to use known donors, too. If this is the case, the sperm will still be checked in the same way and quarantined, and there will also be counselling for both the donor and the recipient to make sure that all the implications have been considered. You should have thought about how much involvement, if any, the donor will have in the child's life and what you will tell them about their conception. Your relationship with the donor is important and you need to talk through all the eventualities and feel as confident as you can that there are not going to be problems further down the line.

Donor eggs

For anyone who has had an early or premature menopause, or for older women whose hormone levels suggest that their ovarian reserve is low, donor eggs may be the answer. Egg donation is quite an involved process, and the woman who is donating will have to take drugs to stimulate her ovaries and have her eggs collected in the same way as anyone else who is going through IVF.

There are shortages of egg donors, and the waiting lists for treatment with donor eggs are often long, which can lead people to seek treatment overseas. In some parts of the world, egg donors are paid and this can attract women who wouldn't otherwise consider donating. It is never easy to recruit altruistic donors, because of the lengthy and intrusive nature of the procedure. Occasionally, friends or family of a woman who needs donor eggs decide that they would be willing to donate. This can be done on a known-donor basis where the woman who needs treatment will use the donated eggs herself. However, in some circumstances, this isn't appropriate and the implications can be complex, so an alternative is to push the woman who has brought the donor along to the top of the waiting list, and to give her donor's eggs to the pool, where they can be offered to whoever is next in line.

Most women are not in a position to bring an egg donor with them to the clinic, and some advertise to try to find someone who might offer. It can be hard to find anyone willing to do this, and even if you do, they may not fit the bill. Clinics don't usually accept donors who are over 35 because treatment using their eggs is less likely to be successful, and anyone who is going to donate will have to go through health checks. These may include tests for any inheritable conditions, as well as HIV and hepatitis. The clinic will also want to make sure that the donor's hormone levels are normal for her age.

Using a donated egg may sound simple, but it can take time to come to terms with it emotionally. Isobel had tried IVF seven times, but every time the treatment had to be abandoned because her body wasn't responding to the drugs. Even so, she had doubts about using donor eggs:

> The strongest feeling for me was that it was second best. Nobody would choose to have a donor-egg baby if they could have their own. One of the big things about wanting a family with my husband was seeing what a little

bit of him and a little bit of me would make, and I felt terribly jealous – I didn't want him to have a child with another woman, which was how I viewed it.

Isobel finally realised that for her this wasn't the second-best choice, but the only choice if she wanted to get pregnant and have a child, but having these doubts and fears is perfectly normal. Nicola had been through unsuccessful IVF, and was having menopausal symptoms, so when doctors suggested donor eggs it was not unexpected, but she says that talking to other people helped her realise that it was natural to have concerns: 'Everyone I've spoken to who has had donor treatment has gone into it having some reservations because it is such a big thing. I think anybody who goes into it saying they are 100 per cent OK with it is probably being naive.'

Trying to sweep your concerns under the carpet and pretend they don't exist is not a good way of dealing with this. There have been cases where women have got pregnant with a donor egg, and have only then faced up to how they feel about it. This has the potential for disaster, and understanding that you are bound to have some qualms and taking time to think about them is by far the best way ahead.

Egg sharing

There has been a growth in the number of clinics offering egg-sharing schemes in recent years, as it is a way around egg shortages. Under these schemes a woman who needs IVF can get cut-price treatment if she offers to share the eggs she produces with another couple who need an egg donor. Not everyone will qualify for this, as you have to be under 35 and healthy, with good hormone levels.

Some people think egg-sharing schemes are unethical, claiming that it is not right for a woman to give away half her eggs just because it is the only way she can afford to have the IVF treatment she needs. Others believe it may be unethical to let women who do not need fertility treatment become altruistic egg donors, as they will have to go through most of an IVF cycle which carries a risk of hyperstimulation (page 84), and at the very least is going to be disruptive and invasive.

Egg sharers take drugs to synchronise their cycles, and after egg collection the eggs will be divided between the two women. Normally, they take half the eggs each, but the situation can become more difficult if the donor produces very few eggs, as then a decision has to be taken as to who should have them. Clinics have their own ways of dealing with these situations, and you need to be clear what these are before you start out.

Surrogacy

Using a surrogate is a complicated and legally challenging route to parenthood, but it has helped many couples who have no other way to have a child of their own. In traditional, or straight, surrogacy, the surrogate will use her own eggs, and either inseminates herself with the intended father's sperm, or has this done at a clinic. The type of surrogacy we are more interested in here is host, or IVF, surrogacy, where the surrogate uses embryos created by both the intended parents or by an egg donor and the intended father. Surrogates may also use embryos created from donated eggs and donated sperm. IVF surrogacy is legally more complicated than traditional surrogacy, but it may make it easier for both the intended parents and the surrogate to cope emotionally. It will be carried out in a clinic and is tightly regulated.

The first surrogate IVF baby was born in the late 1980s, and there has been a slow rise in the number of couples considering IVF surrogacy as people become more aware of the possibility. It is essential for both the surrogate and the intended parents to have proper counselling before entering into a surrogacy arrangement, and to take legal advice.

Some couples travel overseas for surrogacy, as it often appears to be a cheaper and easier option, but if you are considering this, you have to be fully aware of the legal position on surrogacy in both your own country and the country you intend to have treatment in. You should consult a lawyer, as there have been some nightmarish situations where people have used surrogates overseas and ended up in legal wrangles. There have even been reports of intended parents being arrested and children taken into care when overseas surrogacy arrangements have gone wrong.

Surrogacy is not something anyone enters into lightly, and finding someone who is willing to be a surrogate can be a lengthy and time-consuming business. There are helpful support groups for anyone considering or going through surrogacy. There are also some agencies who arrange surrogacy, but you should do your research and check the legal status of any agency before making an appointment, let alone handing over any cash.

Surrogacy isn't easy to come to terms with and if you

have doubts, don't be afraid to admit to them, even if you have already gone some way down the line. Kylie and her partner had spent three years looking for a surrogate and had found someone they liked and trusted, but when they were close to starting treatment, Kylie got cold feet:

> When it came to it, all these emotions came in, which I didn't think were going to be there. You try to suppress them and tell yourself not to be silly, but as it got closer, they were becoming stronger and stronger. I eventually shared them with my husband and he was upset because we'd got this far, but the best thing to do was to be honest – I just didn't know how I was going to feel about someone else carrying my baby.

Kylie has since been for counselling, and has put plans in motion to start the surrogacy process again.

Counselling

Anyone considering using donor sperm, eggs or embryos, or surrogacy, should have counselling before they start. You should be offered implications counselling, where the counsellor will be able to talk through all the short- and long-term consequences of your treatment.

This counselling is often a mandatory part of treatment, and you may discover that you are expected to have it whether you want it or not. Patients sometimes assume this means that the counsellor will be giving them the go-ahead for treatment based on whether they give the right answers to the questions raised during the session. This isn't the case, and Olivia Montuschi of the Donor Conception Network says that you shouldn't just say what you think the counsellor wants to hear:

> Counselling is definitely an opportunity, not a threat. Talking about difficult feelings is sometimes much easier with a third party, particularly with someone like a counsellor whose job it is to listen and not to judge. Any well-qualified counsellor will take the expression of fears as evidence that the couple or individual is taking time to think things through fully, and will be pleased to help them express and explore their feelings, thus helping them make the decision that is right for them.

When Isobel went for counselling before her treatment with donor eggs, she was very worried that the counsellor was judging whether she was suitable for donor treatment based on what she said in the session. She admits she was careful not to raise any of her real feelings or concerns:

> Nobody makes it clear whether the counsellors can veto your treatment or not, so everybody says what they think the counsellors want to hear. I know so many people who have done exactly what we did – just said all the right things: *We've come to terms with it; we are going to tell the children* – all in case the counsellors can stop the cycle.

Counsellors are sometimes aware that patients aren't being truthful, and it is important to be clear about what is going on in this session. The counsellor wants to make sure that you have thought through all the consequences, and is not so concerned with the decisions you have made, but rather with the process you've been through to get to them. They are not looking for specific answers to specific questions, as this counsellor explains:

> When clients go through counselling, it is part of a multi-disciplinary assessment process. They come and they see the doctor and they see the nurse and they see the counsellor and we form an opinion together. There is no point in undergoing counselling if you are going to lie your way through it.

Counselling doesn't suit everyone. If you're someone who doesn't feel comfortable with it, or you don't find it helpful, then you may just have to put up with a session if your clinic requires it. You may find it is more useful than you'd expected, but that can depend on your feelings about the counsellor. Jennifer found this a barrier when she went for implications counselling before using donor sperm:

> We had to have counselling, as it was called. I found the counsellor unbelievably ignorant about all kinds of things, and it was really frustrating to have to sit there, even if it was only for an hour, thinking that your relationship was up for inspection by the hospital and that they were going to be able to say whether you were fit to be a parent or not.

To tell or not to tell

Part of the counselling session will focus on whether you are going to tell your future children about their conception and, if so, what you are going to tell them. As more and more people conceived through donor insemination have reached adulthood, there is an increasing awareness of the potential problems of not telling, particularly in cases where someone who was conceived using donor eggs or sperm finds this out for the first time as an adult, which can be devastating. If any one of your friends or family knows you are having donor treatment, you have to accept that there is a chance your child will find out, whether you decide to tell them or not. Like many working in the field, Olivia Montuschi of the Donor Conception Network feels it is important to be truthful:

> There is plenty of evidence from donor-conceived adults that many of them felt that there was something very odd or wrong in their family, and that this was to do with them. Not having an explanation for this, they blamed themselves. When they discovered they were donor conceived, many felt betrayed and found it difficult to trust their parents afterwards.

Isobel had always imagined she and her husband would keep the fact that they'd used donor eggs a secret from their children, but was surprised to find that her attitude towards this changed when she gave birth: 'While I was pregnant I was insecure about it, and thought I was convinced we would never tell them, but from the first time I saw them, it just didn't seem to matter any more. They were mine.'

Many couples find that they feel this way, and the earlier you tell your children about their conception, the easier it will be. If this is something they have grown up knowing, they will accept it. It's usually only upsetting or awkward if you delay telling children until they are much older.

IVF for single women

The situation has changed considerably for single women who need IVF treatment. Until relatively recently, some clinics simply refused to offer IVF to women who didn't have partners. Now, attitudes have changed, and more single women and lesbian couples are coming forward. They are, however, still a minority, as this nurse explains: 'We've always treated single women and same-sex couples, and we are seeing an increase, but we're seeing an increase in everything else – you're not going to get busloads of single women and lesbians coming up the path, it's just not like that.'

If you have difficulty getting access to treatment, it can make an already difficult situation even tougher, as Annabel found. She'd already had two cycles of IVF with a boyfriend, but when they split up and she decided she wanted to try to have a child by herself, it took some time to find a clinic that would treat her:

I went back to the clinic I'd been to and they said no, they didn't entertain single women, and then I phoned round other clinics and they said the same thing, I had to go to a clinic that was two hours away on the train, and I did find that quite difficult, doing it all on my own.

After a couple of unsuccessful cycles with long journeys involved, she went back to the original clinic and pleaded with them again:

I said it's very difficult emotionally and financially, and I would feel more at ease if I could actually get treatment where I live, I broke down in front of the consultant, and she said the only thing she could do was take it to the ethics committee, and they eventually said they were willing to do it.

IVF can be a lonely process at the best of times, and this is exacerbated if you have to go through the whole thing by yourself. You may not feel able to discuss every nuance of treatment with your friends and family, and this is why a good counsellor can be invaluable if you're going it alone. It is true that many women who have partners go to the clinic alone for some of the scans and blood tests, but their partners will usually be there to support them during the egg collection and embryo transfer, and these can be particularly lonely times. Some single women say they feel clinic staff are less enthusiastic and sympathetic towards them because they are alone, and if you feel this, it may be that you haven't found the right clinic.

Despite all the problems, Annabel says she gets excited each time she has an IVF cycle, because at least there is some hope of achieving her dream:

If you're in a relationship, it might just happen naturally, but when you're in my situation and using donor sperm, this is the only time you've got a bit of hope of falling pregnant. I think you really need to be determined and focused, because if you aren't you will fall apart. For a single person, you really need to have your heart in it, you can't do it on a whim.

IVF for lesbian couples

The problems with access to treatment that can cause difficulty for single women also apply to lesbian couples, and if you are able to find a clinic that has experience treating lesbian couples, it may be far easier for you both. One possible advantage for lesbian couples is that they don't face the same expectations from everyone around them that they are about to reproduce as soon as they've spent a reasonable amount of time together, and this is one of the many difficulties of infertility and IVF that you may be spared. However, some couples find that the prejudices they may encounter on the way more than make up for this.

When Jennifer found she was going to need medical help to conceive, the clinic she went to didn't jump at the idea of treating her:

> They said it had to go to their ethics board. They did finally agree to treat me, but it was made clear to me that I shouldn't talk to the nurses who were actually treating me and that I ought to come across as someone who hadn't had time to have children. That was really humiliating, and hopefully wouldn't happen now.

Travelling abroad for treatment

Couples who need donor treatment are often tempted to travel for their treatment, as donor eggs, sperm and embryos are far more readily available in some parts of the world than in others. In countries where all donors are identifiable, this can reduce the number of people coming forward to donate, but it has on the whole been welcomed by experts, who feel it is important that everyone has a right to trace their genetic parents. Some, like Olivia Montuschi of the Donor Conception Network, urge caution when it comes to travelling for donor treatment:

> I think one of the reasons for the popularity of going abroad is that it feels like being able to take control in a situation. It is convenient for some people that most European countries do not believe in counselling and have completely anonymous donors. It is easy, and understandable, to lose sight of what the child might feel about what you are doing when the focus is very narrowly on becoming pregnant.

You should also be clear about how much information you will get about the donor, how close a match the clinic will be able to offer you, and when you will be able to find this out. There have been reports of couples not being told anything about the donor until they are about to go through embryo transfer. Overseas clinics may not offer follow-up or after care as well as counselling, and things will be much easier if you have the support of a doctor, or a clinic, close to home.

Getting support

When you're using donor sperm or eggs, the isolation and loneliness you feel can become overwhelming. Many of the infertility websites have separate forums for those who are using donor eggs or sperm, and it can be extremely helpful to talk to other people who are going through the same thing. There are also specialist support networks out there waiting to help, and Olivia Montuschi of the Donor Conception Network explains what they can offer:

First and foremost, contact with others in a similar situation — breaking the isolation. Knowing you are not the only person or couple in the world who has had to create their family in this way helps a lot. Sharing stories, finding out how others have faced and managed infertility, donor conception issues and parenting, helps people decide how to move forward and decide how to manage it for themselves.

Chapter twelve

What Can You Do to Make a Difference?

What most of us desperately want to know from the start of our treatment is what we can do to influence the outcome. It's a question I've put to almost everyone I've spoken to at every clinic I've visited, and the initial response has always been exactly the same: a particularly unhelpful 'nothing'. However, most have then gone on to qualify that with one or two tips that may help improve the chances of success, or perhaps just get you through treatment more easily. I've asked patients, too, and I've listed the recommendations below, in the hope that they may of be some help.

Smoking

'Stop smoking – that's the biggie,' an embryologist advised. There is no doubt that smoking has an adverse effect on your fertility. Even back in the very early days of IVF, the patient literature given out by one of the first fertility clinics advised that 'smoking by the wife at any stage of treatment carries the risk that the (embryo) transfer will be a failure'. In those early days, not only were all women going through IVF assumed to be wives, but it also sounds as if their husbands were allowed to carry on smoking as much as they pleased. Now we know that just living with a partner who smokes can mean it will take longer for a woman to get pregnant.

There have been a number of studies linking smoking and sperm problems in men. It is thought that the sperm of smokers have a greater risk of being abnormal, and may be less likely to be able to fertilise an egg. Women who smoke are twice as likely to have fertility problems as non-smokers, and may reach the menopause earlier. One study suggested that smoking could reduce a woman's reproductive life by as much as ten years. The links between smoking and miscarriage, and the dangers smoking can do to an unborn baby, should convince you that it is worth giving up when you are going through IVF.

Alcohol

Some couples give up drinking altogether as soon as they realise they are going to need help to conceive, and there is evidence that heavy drinking can have a detrimental effect on your fertility. Research has found that women who drink more than five units of alcohol a week take longer to get pregnant, and excess or binge drinking may have a negative impact on your menstrual cycle and ovulation, and increase the risk of miscarriage. For men, too, there is evidence that drinking affects sperm.

One consultant said that his key suggestion for men seeking to improve their chances of successful IVF would be to make sure they didn't go on a heavy-drinking stag weekend in the lead-up to treatment.

Here, as with everything else, moderation is the key. If you have an occasional glass of wine, it really isn't going to do any harm. I went to a fortieth birthday party a few days after one embryo transfer and spent the entire evening wandering about holding the same glass of champagne. At one point, during the birthday toast, I allowed myself a sip, and then spent the rest of the night worrying about whether I'd just damaged my chances of getting pregnant. Realistically one sip is not going to make the least bit of difference, but it is easy to start thinking that way when you are trying so hard to do the right thing.

Most clinics advise giving up alcohol completely during the two-week waiting period, and you should follow their advice, at least for this relatively short time. If you are going to find not drinking for a couple of weeks really tough, it may be good for you to give up for a while anyway. Some suggest you should avoid alcohol throughout the entire cycle, whereas others believe you are unlikely to take any risks if you limit yourself to one or two units once or twice a week. One complementary therapist said she had found that giving people mental images of the effects of alcohol helped them visualise why drinking could be a problem: 'If somebody drinks a lot, I'll say to them imagine putting a glass of wine in a baby's bottle, or giving it to a developing sperm. It would have considerably more effect than it would on an adult. I try and explain it in a graphic manner.'

Recreational drugs

It should go without saying that taking any kind of recreational drug when you are trying to conceive is not a good idea. You wouldn't if you were pregnant, so don't when you are trying to get pregnant. Drugs may be a more acceptable part of many social lives than they were 20 years ago, but it isn't worth risking the chance that they may stop your treatment working or damage an unborn baby. Some dope smokers feel that cannabis is harmless and doesn't really count, but it can have a serious impact on both male and female fertility and should be avoided when you are trying to conceive.

Men should also be aware that taking anabolic steroids can shrink your testicles and stop sperm production altogether. Once you stop taking them, the impact on your fertility is usually reversible but this is not always the case if you have been taking high doses for a long period of time.

Weight

Weight can have a huge impact on your chances of getting pregnant, but it is those who are quite significantly overweight or underweight who are going to find that their weight causes problems. Many women feel they could do with losing a few pounds, but being rather rounded, or alternatively slight and slim, is most unlikely to affect your fertility.

There is some evidence that women who are obese are less likely to succeed with IVF, as they may not respond as well to the drugs, and this has led some clinics to refuse treatment to women who they feel are very overweight. Weight is normally assessed by checking your Body Mass Index, or BMI, which is calculated by dividing your weight in kilograms by your height in metres squared. The easiest way to work this out is to type 'BMI calculator' into your search engine on the Internet, and you'll find links to dozens of Web pages where the calculation will be done for you when you type in your height and weight. Generally, a BMI of over 30 is considered to be a potential problem, and if you weigh more than this you may be asked to lose weight before having treatment, as this consultant explains: 'We advise anybody who has a BMI of over 30 to take at least one episode of exercise a week, and if their BMI is over 35 we have concerns about treating them because of response to the medication.'

Losing weight is never easy, but it can be particularly tough when you are unhappy about not being able to get pregnant. This can be a real issue for women who have polycystic ovary syndrome, a fertility problem often linked with being overweight, as it is often harder for them to shed excess pounds. However, as this fertility nurse explains, it is worth making the effort:

Pre-conceptual care is so important, and we have got this big problem with obesity in the population. People say, 'I'm so depressed that I'm not getting pregnant that I am comfort eating,' but you have to have some willpower. We know that if you are very overweight, you have less chance of getting pregnant.

It is important to remember that it is not just women who are very overweight who may have problems with their fertility. Women who are extremely thin, and have a BMI of under 19, may also put their fertility at risk, and they may not respond as well to treatment. When a woman has too little body fat, this can affect the menstrual cycle and stop ovulation.

Diet

You need to make sure you eat properly when you are going through IVF to ensure that your body is getting all the vitamins and nutrients it needs. This will ensure your body is in the best condition for an embryo to implant. Sometimes it can be hard to maintain a healthy diet when you are busy at work and dashing about all the time, but you should try to make an effort, at least during the weeks that you are having treatment. Some clinics suggest that you should make sure you are drinking enough water at this stage, and one clinic I visited advised patients to drink some milk every day, too.

Complementary therapists often advise cutting out caffeine altogether when you're trying to get pregnant, as there have been suggestions that it can reduce your fertility. It does seem that large quantities of caffeine are probably not a good idea at this stage, but the evidence is inconsistent when it comes to the link between caffeine and infertility. You may want to at least limit your caffeine intake during treatment, and remember that it is found in tea and fizzy drinks as well as coffee.

Supplements

Anyone who is trying to get pregnant should be taking folic acid, and you may choose to take a multivitamin. If you have a healthy diet, you shouldn't need to be taking lots of other supplements. In fact, it is not always advisable to take large doses of individual vitamins or supplements, especially if you are combining a number of different substances. If you are planning to take individual supplements during your treatment, you should have a word with the staff at the clinic about it. They may be perfectly happy with this, but sometimes they have concerns about certain supplements and it is worth checking.

Exercise

When one consultant told me the only thing that might make a difference to the outcome of treatment was exercise, I thought he was about to say that everyone should get lots of it. In fact what he said was that women should be careful not to do too much. Women who are devoting hours every day to fitness and exercise may be reducing their fertility, and their chances of a successful outcome from IVF.

However (and yes, there was bound to be a however here), this does only apply to quite serious fitness training, and is not likely to be a problem for the majority of women. You need some exercise if you are going to lead a healthy lifestyle, and it can have a significant impact on reducing stress and increasing your sense of well-being.

Moderate exercise is more likely to have a positive effect on the outcome of your treatment.

Stress

Most of us worry about our stress levels when we are going through IVF treatment, and although there is some conflicting evidence as to what effect it may have on the outcome of treatment, most of the medical professionals I spoke to did feel it could make a difference, as this consultant explained: 'There is a large body of evidence to suggest that stress is detrimental to reproductive function, and that it might to some extent compromise the outcome of treatment.'

When I was trying to get pregnant, I always found that the more I worried about my stress levels, the more stressed I felt. Most of us have probably been advised to 'relax and it will happen' at some point on our fertility journeys, but people forget that not being able to conceive is a cause of stress in itself. It can start to feel like a vicious circle: your fertility problems make you stressed, and then the stress you feel makes you less likely to overcome the fertility problems that made you stressed in the first place . . .

You may not be able to eliminate the stress caused by infertility, but you can do something about the other stressful elements of your life, as this consultant suggests:

We always say reduce your stress levels. It's amazing how many people decide to move house during fertility treatment, to do two of the most stressful things you can do

in life at the same time. One of them can wait for another
month. Then you will be in a better position to feel well and
able to cope, rather than uptight and worried.

As someone who moved house the day before egg collection, I am guilty here. I certainly wouldn't recommend it,
although for me the combination of moving house and
IVF was less stressful than going to work and IVF during
the early part of the treatment, and in fact, this was the
cycle that worked for us. Perhaps what it proves is that
causes of stress are very personal. If there is something in
your life that is making you anxious and worried, try to
reduce your exposure to it when you are having IVF.

Lifestyle

'I think the only thing a couple can do is maintain a
healthy lifestyle,' one consultant told me. Since you are
likely to have spent considerable amounts of time and
money on IVF, it does make sense to try to optimise your
chances of success by making sure you are as fit and
healthy as you can be when you have treatment.

It's a sentiment echoed by one of the nurses I spoke
to, who felt that in purely financial terms it was worth
making sure you'd done all you could to help: 'It is defin-
itely worth investing in your lifestyle before you start
paying for fertility treatment, because so much rides on
it,' she said. 'If you smoke or drink too much, you are
not doing your bank account any favours by not giving
yourself the best possible chance.' For most people, a few
simple improvements will be all that is needed, and it

is only those who have particularly unhealthy lifestyles who will find they need to make radical changes.

Your attitude

Most medical professionals agree that some couples seem to cope with the experience far better than others, but none can pinpoint exactly what this comes down to. It may be related to stress and lifestyle, or it may be just different personality types.

Najeeb and his partner had four IVF cycles before their treatment worked, and they tried not to focus on possible outcomes:

> It was a project. We used to try and visualise it as a technical problem for which we needed to find a solution. We took away the emotional view of the future we had in the first cycle, where you were thinking, *in nine months we are going to have a baby.* Our mission was much more short term, and we took it one step at a time rather than looking at the end result of carrying around a baby.

It's unrealistic to suggest that you should stop thinking about possible outcomes, and success or failure, but if you can try to take each step of treatment at a time, and focus on reaching the next goal along the way, you may find that it makes it easier to cope. People who manage to do this, do seem to stay calmer, but it can be hard to implement this approach successfully.

Complementary therapies

Although complementary therapies aren't for everyone, they may help you to feel calmer and more relaxed during treatment, and you will find more information about individual therapies in the next chapter.

Finding out as much as you can

When I asked people who had been through IVF what they felt made a difference, most of them said that they'd advise people to find out all they could about treatment, to read all they could, and particularly to try to learn about other people's experiences of IVF through support groups, books and magazines or on the Internet.

Looking after yourself

Another tip from patients was to make sure that you make some time to do the things you enjoy, and to treat yourself. When you're so focused on treatment, it can be hard to remember to do this, but it is important. For some people relaxing and enjoying themselves had meant a weekend away, or a day at a spa, for others it was joining a yoga class or an evening out at a restaurant every now and again. These can be simple things, but remember that IVF is never easy, and if you can spoil yourself every now and again, you should take the opportunity.

The weird ones

Own up if you're wearing orange knickers? Or going to bed at night with a hot water bottle on your tummy? Have you been buying special 'fertility jewellery' online? Do you have a picture of a pomegranate on your bedroom wall? Or a set of seven elephants on your bedside table? Do you own an African fertility doll or a small ceramic fertility frog? Have you jumped over a bonfire on the night of the summer solstice? Or dragged your partner up to the Cerne Abbas Giant in Dorset? Do you carry a bag of hazelnuts around with you? If you answered no to every one of those, don't worry. I'm pleased to tell you it won't make the least difference to your chances of having a baby.

There are some peculiar myths, traditions and rituals around infertility, and when nothing else seems to work, it can be tempting to try them. Even the most logical, rational people may find themselves doing things, or buying things, they know can't really make a difference, but convince themselves that if it isn't going to do any harm it may be worth a try.

I will admit at this point that I stopped walking under ladders when I was going through my fertility treatment. I also developed a strange obsession with counting magpies ('one for sorrow, two for joy, three for a girl, four for a boy'). It's amazing how unusual it is to see three or four, or even two, magpies together when you want to, but I used to feel this strange surge of hope whenever I happened to notice a group of them pecking about.

It wasn't just me; perfectly sane friends and family members would draw me aside and whisper in slightly embarrassed tones that they had something that might help, and that's how I ended up with a fertility doll from Africa, a witches' charm and a framed photo of an ancient fertility shrine in Greece where a blessing was made on my behalf. I was touched that other people had understood how we were feeling, and had gone to so much trouble to try to find something that they thought might possibly help, or at least make me feel better.

Most of these fertility aids aren't going to do any harm, but don't expect them to do any good either. There are people making a lot of money selling all kinds of stuff that you wouldn't buy in a more rational mood. If you happen to have a penchant for ceramic frogs, or pictures of pomegranates, that's fine, but don't get swept into thinking that if you don't buy them, your treatment is less likely to work. Of course, some women wearing orange knickers are going to get pregnant, but so are lots of others wearing white, or blue, or black ones.

Don't worry

Perhaps the bottom line on all this is don't panic. The majority of people manage to conceive without following special diets or exercise regimes, and once your fertilised embryo has been put back into the womb, you should be able to get on with your life as normal. Don't be too hard on yourself, or have unrealistic expectations of the perfect lifestyle you ought to be leading. Ultimately, as long as you are sensible and try to keep healthy, you are doing the best you can to help, and getting stressed and guilty about what you're doing or not doing is certainly not going to improve the situation.

Chapter thirteen

Complementary Therapies and IVF

Complementary therapies are increasingly popular for all kinds of ailments and illnesses, and there are a multitude of practitioners claiming to have produced miracle babies for couples with fertility problems. Although there may be anecdotal evidence from satisfied customers, there is scant scientific proof to back up any of these claims, and it can be hard to know what to believe.

Many complementary therapies take a holistic approach, and work on treating both your mind and body. The treatments tend to be relaxing, and can enhance your feelings of well-being. There is usually time to talk to the therapist, and an element of counselling which can have positive effects on how you feel about your treatment and your situation. People often find that the relaxation and counselling element of these therapies are particularly helpful.

The medical point of view

Doctors are traditionally sceptical about the whole field of complementary medicine, and if you ask the medical team treating you about complementary therapies, you may get a distinctly lukewarm response. 'To be honest, I don't recommend complementary therapies,' one consultant told me. 'That's mainly because I don't know very much about non-medical treatments. If people find it helpful for themselves, I'm not aware of any disadvantages.'

Others were worried that in some circumstances complementary therapies could cause problems:

> Our concern would be that we couldn't be sure it was actually complementary to what we were doing. If we are trying to down-regulate a patient, how do we know that the complementary therapist is also trying to down-regulate them? Or say they were trying to stimulate the ovaries with complementary medicine that might be contra-indicated by whatever we were trying to do in their treatment.

Perhaps the best solution is to tell your doctor if you are having complementary therapies during IVF, and to make sure your complementary therapist is aware of everything that is happening in your conventional treatment. Doctors will not usually have problems with patients getting help outside the clinic if it helps them cope. There are even some clinics that work with complementary therapists who come into the unit and treat patients there, but this kind of joint treatment venture is far from widespread.

Therapies that may help

Choosing a complementary therapy is not like choosing a fertility clinic where you will be able to look at success rates and make a balanced judgement. This is a more personal matter of choosing something that has the potential to help you relax and a therapist you can feel comfortable with, and have confidence in. You may want to ask whether a therapist has experience with couples with fertility problems, or those who are going through IVF.

You should think about the cost of treatment, too. If your budget is tight, you won't want to shell out for an individualised treatment package at a holistic therapy centre where you might be paying for a variety of treatments, tonics and supplements. Before agreeing to any complementary therapy, you should make sure that the practitioner you are seeing is properly qualified and registered with the appropriate regulatory or governing body. There is a list of these at the end of the book, and many have websites that will enable you to find a recommended practitioner in your area.

Acupuncture

This traditional Chinese treatment dates back thousands of years, and it is one of the most widely used complementary therapies for infertility. There has been some research to suggest that acupuncture may help boost the chances of a successful outcome if it is used around the time of embryo transfer during IVF, and this has made it more popular with fertility patients. However, the evidence is far from clear on this. Another study that looked at all the available evidence on the subject found that there was no link at all between acupuncture and increased IVF success.

Some men and women do say acupuncture has made them feel better even if it didn't necessarily help them conceive, and this acupuncturist believes the calming effect of the therapy can help during IVF:

> Acupuncture can really calm the patient down, and if you do something that can calm the system, it can give the fertilised embryo more chance of implanting. Also, after implantation, if you are really calm and not excessively worried or stressed, that can help prevent miscarriage as well. That is why so many patients like to have acupuncture before and after the transfer.

Although many people do feel acupuncture has a calming effect, there is conflicting evidence about this, too, and the research on the subject is far from conclusive.

Acupuncture involves sticking thin needles through the skin at specific points in the body, and this is meant to help balance the flow of our life force, qi (pronounced 'chee'), around our bodies. It is believed that the qi passes around the body in invisible pathways called meridians, and that these can become blocked. Acupuncture aims to try to balance the two natural forces that control our bodies, the yin and yang, as imbalances are thought to cause illness.

The acupuncturist will spend some time talking to you before any needles are involved, and you may be asked questions about different aspects of your life and your feelings about your infertility. The acupuncturist will feel your pulse, as they detect more about possible imbalances this way, and look at your tongue. They may make some dietary recommendations, advising that you should avoid certain foods and eat more of others.

It is a holistic approach, and the acupuncturist will not be treating you for the particular cause of your infertility, but rather trying to balance your entire body. This acupuncturist explains the philosophy and how it can help:

> We treat the body as a whole, and a healthy body depends on a balance of all the internal organs. If any one part is out of balance, you will get problems. With IVF there is a lot of stress, and people pay a lot and have to put a lot of hormones in their body. If before you start you can have at least three months of acupuncture or Chinese medicine, it will give you a healthy body to prepare for the IVF.

There's quite a lot of focus on whether acupuncture can help improve the outcome of IVF for women, but it's important not to forget that many people believe it can be just as important in helping male infertility. Najeeb's partner had acupuncture before and during IVF, and he went for a regular course of treatment, too:

> There is no hard medical proof, but I did feel it had far-reaching health benefits for me. I had weekly treatments and over a six-month period with the change of diet, cutting out drinking and the extra fitness, it enabled me to more than double my sperm count, which was good from a clinical point of view, but also good from an emotional point of view, because it made us feel we were going to do better.

Traditional Chinese medicine

Acupuncture is just one branch of the treatments offered in traditional Chinese medicine, and an acupuncturist may also prescribe herbal remedies. Traditionally, the herbal remedies were given as dried herbs that were used to make tea, but now they sometimes come in freeze-dried formulas, too, which are easier and less time-consuming to take. People who are not used to taking Chinese herbal formulas often find the taste quite unpleasant at first, but apparently you do get used to them after a while. Although more IVF patients are now using herbs along with acupuncture, this is a less well-known part of Chinese medicine, as this practitioner explains: 'People only know about acupuncture, but they don't know about the whole picture behind that. Acupuncture can open the energy channels, but if the person has an underlying problem, that will depend on the herbs, which can work on the whole system.'

Conventional doctors sometimes have concerns about traditional Chinese medicine, as it is not always clear what the herbal remedies contain and some have pharmaceutically active components. Some herbs can be toxic if they are taken in large quantities, and it is vital to ensure you are seeing a properly qualified practitioner. You should check with your fertility clinic that they are happy for you to take these herbal remedies during your treatment.

Herbal medicine

The use of herbs in medicine is not unique to China. People have been using herbs to try to cure illnesses and ailments for centuries, and some of the conventional medicines we use today are made with chemicals derived from herbs. You can buy herbal remedies over the counter in many health-food outlets, but it is worth seeing a qualified herbalist and explaining that you are having fertility treatment before you start taking anything, as some of these remedies may not be right to take at certain times during a treatment cycle.

Herbal medicines are made using the entire plant rather than concentrating on the active chemical compounds. They are often prescribed for female fertility problems such as menstrual irregularity, and claim particular success at dealing with stress and anxiety, which may be useful when you are going through IVF.

Reflexology

Another popular therapy with couples going through fertility treatment, reflexology is based on the idea that specific areas of your feet correspond to particular parts of your body, and that massaging the feet can help with problems throughout the body. It is sometimes suggested that reflexology is an ancient Egyptian or Chinese treatment, but in fact the mapping out of specific zones in the feet relating to particular parts of the body originated in the United States in the 1930s.

Most reflexology sessions last about an hour, and you will begin with a discussion about the nature of the problem before the reflexologist gets to work on your feet. One reflexologist, who specialises in working with couples with fertility problems, explains what happens during a reflexology session:

It's not a massage, it's actually a creeping movement with the thumb. You're doing a little caterpillar walk all over each specific area, and each specific area has a reflex part in the body, so there is a foot map that we work to. The whole of the feet are like a map of the whole of the body.

The reflexologist says that she can feel with her fingers and thumbs if something is wrong, and can identify where problems are in the body. This doesn't mean that she can always diagnose the problem, as she explains: 'By feeling it I don't necessarily know what's wrong with them but if that area shows tenderness then it might show that their body is out of balance in some way – and you'd do the same treatment whatever the problem, as you are re-balancing the body.'

This re-balancing is not the only way that reflexologists believe they can help. Many people find reflexology very relaxing, and this reflexologist feels it gives them a better chance of getting pregnant:

> People are often not very good at relaxing, and the fact that they are coming once a week for an hour means they completely de-stress about their problems and relax. That goes an awfully long way to help balancing the body up. Stress causes all sorts of havoc in the body. If you reduce all that and keep the body calmer, then that is going to help.

Emma went to see a reflexologist in the run up to her treatment, and she believes it did make a difference:

> I did reflexology both times, and I'd certainly be inclined to try it again, because it got me pregnant both times. You can't do it once you've started the treatment but I did it

leading up to starting the drugs. It did help me relax and it was the one time I had to lie down for an hour and I couldn't rush around doing things.

If you're going to have reflexology to help you get through your IVF treatment, therapists would recommend you start the reflexology about three months before you begin, and try to have a treatment every week. Reflexology is not always recommended in early pregnancy, and although some practitioners are happy to treat people who are in the first few months of pregnancy, others are not. This means that reflexology may not be a suitable treatment once you have started the IVF cycle, and you may want to think about another kind of complementary therapy if your reflexologist is not happy to do a session at this time.

Aromatherapy

This treatment involves the use of essential oils, which are usually massaged into the body. The oils are extracted from plants, and often have quite strong scents. They are diluted into a carrier or base oil before they are used for massage. Oils can also be used in the bath, or in an oil burner, so that you can inhale the scent.

It isn't entirely clear how the aromatherapy oils affect the body, but the pleasant smell and the relaxing nature of the massage can be very calming. You should make sure your practitioner knows you are having IVF, as there are some oils that must not be used during early pregnancy.

Homeopathy

The homeopath focuses on the whole body rather than individual symptoms, as it is thought that your emotional and psychological health may play a significant role in illness, which is often caused by some kind of imbalance. Homeopathy is based on the theory that 'like cures like', and a homeopath will prescribe tiny doses of substances that can produce the symptoms of an illness in order to cure the illness itself.

Homeopathic medicines can be derived from plant, mineral or animal sources, but they are heavily diluted before being made into pills or powders. It is believed that the more dilute the medicine is, the more powerful the effects will be. The remedies can be given in water, or as a small sugar pill. When you take them, you are not meant to eat or drink immediately before or afterwards.

When you visit a homeopath, the consultation will focus on your emotional and psychological well-being as well as your physical symptoms. Your temperament and the way you deal with things are also believed to be relevant. Anyone seeing a homeopath for help with infertility may benefit from this opportunity to explore their feelings about what is happening, and this homeopath recommends starting well before the IVF cycle begins:

I would recommend a couple look at a constitutional treatment for about three months before they start the IVF. That gives them some time to get their general health in good shape. When you give a constitutional remedy, it often makes people more fertile than they were before, now that their body is functioning better. Homeopathy can make you healthier, and increase your chances of getting pregnant.

Homeopaths can prescribe specific remedies to help with some fertility problems, for example to regulate and stimulate ovulation. When it comes to IVF, some homeopaths may prefer not to carry on treating you during the cycle itself, but this will depend on your practitioner. There are others who have a special interest in infertility, and who are happy to work with patients throughout the cycle, as this homeopath explains: 'During the IVF, I try not to interfere with the process at all, as the procedures are very particular. I give a remedy to give reassurance and to soothe the nervous system, and try to support them.'

Lulu feels homeopathy made a difference when she was going through IVF:

I was seeing a homeopath who had lots of experience with infertility, and she put me on a very specific homeopathic programme with pills to take at certain times to help deal with the effects of the drugs, and also to help support the ovaries and to help with implantation. I found it very useful, and I am sure it helped.

Hypnotherapy

The role of stress in infertility has been much discussed, and hypnotherapy aims to help people relax while also resolving any hidden fears or anxieties that may be lurking in the subconscious mind and preventing conception. We often think that being hypnotised means being sent to sleep, but in fact it involves the body being put into a deeply relaxed state so that you are able to make contact with your subconscious.

Hypnosis has been given rather a bad press by hypnotists who take their art to the stage, and get members of the public to make fools of themselves. This has made some people wary of using hypnosis for therapy, but the hypnotherapist I spoke to was keen to explain that there is no need to be worried:

> You can only be hypnotised if you want to be hypnotised – it's as simple as that. Everybody I work with wants to be hypnotised, so they will always go into hypnosis. Some people are a little bit more resistant than others, but that is usually due to the fear of hypnosis itself. I find once I've explained it to them and take them through the process very gently, they are absolutely fine.

There are a number of hypnotherapists who specialise in dealing with fertility problems, and you may be able to find a hypnofertility therapist who has particular expertise in this area. Hypnotherapists aim to help you go into treatment in a more relaxed state, aware of what will be involved and having visualised how you may deal with it.

A hypnotherapy session will begin with a consultation, going through your medical and personal history, and hypnosis will be explained so that you understand that you will be in control of what will happen. If you want to use hypnotherapy to help during IVF, you are advised to start a few months before the cycle, to gain the maximum benefit.

Hypnotherapy is about more than relaxation. Hypnotherapists say they sometimes uncover underlying anxieties that could be playing a role in preventing pregnancy. 'If women have had horrible things happen to them, and don't have a good relationship with the sexual part of themselves we can help release this,' a hypnotherapist explains. 'Past abuse, abortion and guilt can have a huge impact. Also I come across so many women who have been trying so hard to get pregnant that they completely lose faith in their bodies, and don't actually believe they can get pregnant.' Hypnosis aims to calm the underlying fears, and to restore women's belief in their own bodies.

Craniosacral therapy

Developed by an American osteopath in the 1900s, craniosacral therapy involves the therapist lightly touching your body with his or her hands. It is based on the idea that there are subtle rhythms in our bodies that are linked with our well-being, and the therapist 'listens' to these with his or her hands.

These rhythms are thought to be linked to the cerebrospinal fluid, which flows around the brain and spinal cord. The light touching of the therapist apparently adjusts any restrictions or blockages in the flow of the fluid, while also increasing general energy levels and relieving stress. It is perhaps in this stress-relieving role that craniosacral therapy might be useful when you are going through IVF, although some therapists also believe it can help with implantation after embryo transfer.

Bach flower remedies

These remedies are derived from plants and flowers, and were discovered by an English doctor, Edward Bach, in the 1930s. He'd had traditional medical training, and spent many years working in conventional medicine before becoming increasingly convinced that there was too much focus on the illness, and too little on the individual. He identified a number of remedies each aimed at helping with a particular mental state, and Bach flower practitioners focus on dealing with the emotions.

Bach flower remedies are often used by those going through IVF in an attempt to reduce stress and anxiety levels. Aspen is commonly prescribed, as it helps with anxiety, but although it is possible to purchase individual remedies over the counter, therapists say this can be a waste of time and money if you don't know what you are doing. If you visit a trained practitioner, they will make you an individual remedy based on your needs and circumstances that may contain six or seven different essences, and you take drops of the remedy at least four times a day.

Reiki

This is a fairly new healing method, developed in Japan about 100 years ago. The Japanese word reiki means 'universal life energy', and practitioners claim to be able to channel this to help others. In order to be able to use reiki, you have to be initiated, or attuned, into the energy by a reiki master. Once you have been initiated, you can pass the energy on to others.

In a session of reiki, the practitioner places their hands on, or just above, your body in a series of sequences that are meant to remove blockages in your energy flow and get rid of toxins. It is claimed that reiki can help smooth out stressful emotions, and can accelerate natural healing processes. If reiki makes you feel more relaxed and positive, it may well help you through treatment, as this practitioner explains:

> Reiki is a calming relaxing treatment and it works on the emotional and physical level. If people have lots of doubts and don't think pregnancy is ever going to happen for them, it can help them relax and feel that if it is going to happen, let it be now. People do say they find it quite a powerful thing – they say they never thought they'd feel anything, but they feel tingling going down their body and all sorts of things.

Yoga

It may be more a form of exercise than a complementary therapy in the traditional sense, but people often turn to yoga when they are trying unsuccessfully to get pregnant or are going through treatment. Yoga can certainly alleviate stress, and the focus on breathing during yoga classes will help you to feel calm and relaxed. It is also claimed that it may rebalance hormones, increase the blood flow to your reproductive organs and stimulate the ovaries, but the stress-reducing benefits may be particularly helpful to anyone going through an IVF cycle.

Nutritional therapy

Many complementary therapy clinics have a nutritionist on their books. They advise on the best nutrition for conception, and can help make sure that you have all the essential vitamins and minerals your body needs for conception. Sometimes this may be mainly a matter of advising on your diet, which can be helpful and useful.

However, some nutritionists also like to carry out a range of tests, including hair analysis, and will prescribe supplements to make sure your body has all it needs.

Holistic fertility care

Centres offering a range of complementary therapies and supplements specifically designed to help couples with fertility problems seem to be growing in popularity, and you may find a variety of different places offering a whole host of solutions. Some of these clinics are essentially a group of complementary therapists working together under the fertility umbrella at one location. There is often a focus on nutritional advice, and the clinic may suggest that you should be taking dietary supplements. There are other companies offering supplements online, or postal analyses of hair samples.

You could spend most of your time, and vast amounts of money, on the wide variety of treatments, supplements, tinctures and oils offered by holistic fertility centres, and it may be helpful to decide in advance how much you can afford to spend. Otherwise, it is often tempting to keep splashing out in search of the one thing that might make a difference.

A note of caution

It is undoubtedly true that many of these treatments may help you relax and reduce your stress levels, but it is important to be clear about the benefits you could expect. When Clare miscarried for a second time, she thought complementary therapies might have something to offer and went to see a naturopath, but pulled out of the treatment after the therapist began making unrealistic claims for her herbal remedies:

> The naturopath started telling me that if she gave me certain herbs for a certain amount of money, it would unblock my tubes. That's when I started getting very cynical about what she was telling me. She told me all this stuff about my hormone levels being too high at this point of my cycle and too low at this point, which was why I was miscarrying. When I spoke to my consultant about it she said it was absolute rubbish.

Medical professionals do have concerns about claims like these, and about some of the types of treatment and analysis on offer. It is quite common for these complementary therapists to suggest that patients may have vitamin or mineral deficiencies which are causing fertility problems, but the vast majority of us, and particularly those who have the money to visit complementary therapists, are well nourished and unlikely to be suffering from any serious deficiencies. Despite some concerns, most would agree complementary therapies may have a role to play as long as you go into it with a degree of caution. 'I do worry about some of the companies who offer hair analysis and things,' a fertility nurse confessed, 'but if complementary treatments are reasonably priced and are going to help somebody relax and cope with the stress of treatment, then go for what works.'

Men and complementary therapies

All the complementary therapists I've spoken to say they see far more women with fertility problems than men in their clinics. This is partly because the women will be going through the treatment, and perhaps feel they have a greater investment in keeping their bodies in the best condition they can at this time, but it may also reflect the reluctance men often feel about discussing their fertility problems. The therapists say this can make their job more difficult, because infertility is a joint problem and yet, as this homeopath explains, they are only treating half of it:

> I see very few men, and I think it's sad. It could be a male pride thing. Women are more driven, and it is them that are going to have the procedures carried out on them, but I say to them, just tell your partners to come once. If they don't like it, they don't have to come again, but it gives me the opportunity to give them a remedy.

Cost of complementary therapies

You could easily squander a small fortune on complementary therapies, and some people spend as much on alternative therapists as they do at their fertility clinic. If you have the money to spare and it makes you feel better, that's not a problem, but it is important not to get swept along into thinking that if you don't have the cash for complementary treatments, you are putting your chances of successful IVF in jeopardy.

Many of the real benefits of complementary treatments are to do with the relaxation that they can induce, and you may find that you can achieve some of this in other, far less expensive, ways. As this nurse explains:

I would never say to people not to do it, but it is a hell of an expense. When you're scanning people they will sometimes say, 'I've just been to my acupuncturist, it is costing me four hundred pounds a month,' and you do wonder if the stress of the financial ramifications might outweigh the benefits.

Chapter fourteen

When Treatment Doesn't Work

The pregnancy test is the point you've been heading towards, not just through the drugs and scans and IVF itself, but going right back through the years of not getting pregnant that have led you there. So much has been invested in this, and it is an emotional moment.

Home testing

Your clinic may suggest that you use a home pregnancy testing kit, and tell you when you should do this. Alternatively, some clinics will call you in for a blood test, although you may prefer to do your own test at home anyway, rather than waiting for the clinic to tell you whether the treatment has worked or not. Home testing kits are widely available, and on sale in pharmacies and in some supermarkets. There are lots of different brands, and your clinic can probably suggest one that they have found to be reliable.

Most kits are easy to use and come with clear instructions that you should follow carefully. They work by testing for hCG, or human chorionic gonadotrophin, in your urine, and although the tests have become more sensitive in recent years, it is still possible to get a false negative result in very early pregnancy.

Blood test

Some clinics will want you to have a blood test to check whether the treatment has worked, as this is more sensitive and can measure the exact levels of hCG in your body. You may be asked to do a blood test even if your period has already started, as you can have light spotting and still be pregnant. Bleeding could also indicate an ectopic pregnancy (page 226), which would require immediate medical attention.

A blood test can give a more accurate picture of what is happening, and how things are progressing. Doctors sometimes like to do blood tests because your hormone levels will give an idea whether you are likely to be pregnant with twins or a single baby, and can also alert them to a possible ectopic pregnancy.

A low positive result

It is possible for an embryo to implant in the womb, and then stop growing, or to miscarry very early. This is why clinics carry out a scan at around six or seven weeks, to check that they can see a heartbeat. If you have a blood test at the clinic, they may detect what they refer to as a 'low positive'. This means that you have some pregnancy hormones in your blood, but the levels are lower than would be expected.

This can be a difficult outcome to deal with, as you just have to wait and see whether the hormone levels will increase. Sometimes this does happen, and the pregnancy progresses as normal, but in other cases the hormone levels will drop and an early pregnancy will be lost.

The negative test

After all the emotional and financial investment in your treatment, a negative result is devastating, and it can take time for you to come to terms with this. Often neither the doctors nor the embryologists are able to give any reasons why the treatment hasn't worked, and people can end up feeling that it is somehow their fault. If this happens, you should try to remember that it is the treatment that has failed, and not you.

An individual IVF cycle is more likely to be unsuccessful than it is to result in a pregnancy, but knowing this doesn't make it any easier when it is your treatment cycle. You have put so much into the treatment, and you may feel that your emotional stamina has reached an all-time low. I found it took a couple of days for the reality to sink in when our first IVF cycle didn't work. Having initially thought I was coping with it all remarkably well, I suddenly sunk into the depths of despair. I couldn't talk about the IVF, babies or any vaguely related topic without bursting into tears, and I didn't imagine I'd ever have the strength to start again.

If you've told people exactly when you're doing IVF, you may find you wish you hadn't when it gets to this point, as they will all be waiting to know the outcome. Having to tell other people it hasn't worked can be pretty tough. It's a difficult balance because you may want support during the treatment itself, but the other side of this is that they are all going to want to know whether it has worked, and you are going to have to deal with that.

Debbie always told her friends and family when she was having IVF, and felt the benefits of their support outweighed the difficulty of having to tell them when it was unsuccessful:

It's really hard every time you have a negative. It's horrible having to make sure that 20 people know that it hasn't worked, but that's just added on to the pain you are suffering anyway. For me, it would have made the stress so much harder to have kept that to myself and not opened my mouth when people wonder why you look so miserable.

Miscarriage

It's hard enough to lose a baby when you've got pregnant easily, but when it happens after a long period of infertility and IVF, it is devastating. Having allowed yourself to start to feel excited about finally being pregnant only to have that all whisked away feels so cruel.

It can be hugely frustrating if you've had a miscarriage

to discover that no one can give you any clues as to why it might have happened. Miscarriage is far more common than we think, and doctors don't usually investigate the possible causes unless you've had recurrent miscarriages. The idea that no one is going to be particularly interested in finding out what went wrong unless the same thing happens two or three times can seem unbearable, but it is partly because early pregnancy loss does occur so often, and partly because the majority of women who have lost a baby will go on to have a normal pregnancy afterwards.

Helena had already had one miscarriage when she found out she was pregnant after an ICSI cycle: 'I got to seven weeks and there was a heartbeat, but at nine weeks it had stopped. I had lots of tests, but they couldn't find any reason, they didn't find anything wrong. They didn't know why we weren't getting pregnant easily or why I was miscarrying.'

The risk of miscarriage is slightly higher after IVF, but there are some reasons for this. When you've had treatment, you know you are pregnant far earlier than most other people, and women who get pregnant naturally may not be aware of a very early pregnancy loss. The fact that women who have IVF tend to be older may play a role here, as older women have a greater risk of miscarriage, whether they've had help to get pregnant or not. If a woman gets pregnant at 40, she has a 40 per cent risk of having a miscarriage, and by the age of 45 this has risen to 80 per cent. The reason for this age-related increase in miscarriage is probably partly due to some kind of chromosomal abnormality in the fertilised egg. Women with certain fertility problems are also at greater risk, as polycystic ovary syndrome and some hormonal problems have been linked to miscarriage.

There are any number of other possible causes of miscarriage that have nothing to do with infertility or treatment. They include problems with the immune system, infections or the presence of antibodies that can cause blood clots or adverse reactions. Sometimes a weakness in the cervix can lead to a later miscarriage, or it might be caused by abnormalities in the womb itself. Women who smoke increase their chances of losing a baby.

Many people find it helps to try to get some of the emotion they feel after a miscarriage out into the open, and talking about things is useful. You may find that discussing how you feel with your friends or your partner gives you all the time you need for this. It isn't always easy to be frank about your feelings with people you know, however, and seeing a counsellor might help. When Clare had a miscarriage after treatment, she and her partner went to see a counsellor recommended by their clinic: 'We had counselling after the miscarriage – a lot of counselling because we had a lot of things to come to terms with. The counsellor was absolutely brilliant, and I found it hugely helpful.'

Launching into the whole IVF process again after losing a baby is tough, and you are bound to approach it with some trepidation. Sometimes having been pregnant in the past can give hope for the future, as Emma explains: 'Because I had got pregnant, I was trying to cling on to that hope. Obviously, after a miscarriage you have to wait before you can start trying again, so we went on holiday, but I was keen to get on with it again.'

Ectopic pregnancy

If a fertilised embryo implants outside the womb cavity, this is known as an ectopic pregnancy and the embryo will not be able to grow and develop. Although during IVF embryos are transferred into the womb, it is still possible for them to move about and implant elsewhere. Most ectopic pregnancies occur when an embryo implants in the fallopian tube.

If you've had a previous ectopic pregnancy, there is an increased risk of this happening again, and women who have blocked or damaged fallopian tubes are also more likely to have an ectopic. The chances of having an ectopic pregnancy after IVF are slightly higher than for those who get pregnant naturally, but this is likely to be because so many women who have IVF have problems with their fallopian tubes.

The signs of an ectopic pregnancy are pain in the abdomen and bleeding. The bleeding is usually not the same as your normal period, and there may be spotting or it can be dark, watery blood. Some women experience shoulder pain, which is caused by internal bleeding. There may also be bladder or bowel pain. You can feel nauseous and faint, or light-headed.

A pregnancy test will usually show a positive result, although you may need a test at the clinic to pick this up. If your clinic has done a blood test to check whether the treatment has worked, this can sometimes give them an indication that a pregnancy may be ectopic. Otherwise, if you have the signs of an ectopic pregnancy, it is important to get it checked out. Doctors will usually do a pregnancy test and an ultrasound scan.

You may just be monitored for a few days if you have a suspected ectopic pregnancy, and if it is diagnosed early it can sometimes be treated without damaging the tube. For more advanced cases, it is often necessary to remove the fallopian tube completely. This may seem extreme but if the ectopic is allowed to continue to grow, it may cause the fallopian tube to burst and this can be fatal. An ectopic pregnancy is never going to be viable, and it is important to act quickly if there is any possibility that it is going to rupture the tube.

If you have an ectopic pregnancy, you will probably be advised to wait for a while to give your body time to heal before trying IVF again. The emotional after-effects of an ectopic pregnancy can take time to get over, as it is a traumatic experience.

Trying again after a negative result

Some people feel they want to have another go at IVF as soon as they've had a negative test result, but your clinic will usually recommend that you leave some time between cycles, as IVF is a taxing business. For others, the thought of having to go through it all again can seem unbearable, and you may doubt that you'll ever have the strength for another attempt. Once is enough for some people, and they won't ever do it again. For many others, the pain of an unsuccessful attempt does fade slowly, and once they've had some time to get themselves back together again, they may find that they are ready for another go. Having a break from treatment is often a good idea, and if you agree that you won't try again for a specific period, you may benefit from a bit of breathing space.

We all secretly hope that we will be one of the lucky ones who gets pregnant first time around, but most people who have been successful with IVF won't have got pregnant the first time they tried. I heard a consultant talking about cumulative success rates for IVF at a conference recently, and he explained that although we think of it as a relatively unsuccessful treatment, the chances of success do improve for couples who have the strength and the finances to keep going. He made the point that when people are trying to get pregnant naturally, they don't expect it to work in the very first month, and that they wouldn't give up if it hadn't worked after the second or third month either. Of course it is very different for IVF patients, as there's often a limit to how much they can take and how much they can afford, but it is true that some people who can keep going, do get pregnant eventually. Unfortunately, others who have many attempts still won't succeed, and there are no guarantees. There are cases of couples who finally have a child after 15 or more unsuccessful attempts at IVF, but not many of us would have the money or the stamina to keep going for that long. What makes it so difficult is that there is no certainty you will ever be one of the lucky ones, however many times you try.

Alison, who has stopped having IVF, says there was pressure to keep going because people assume that if you keep trying, it must work eventually:

The world only hears of the successes. When you talk to people about it, they push you to do it again – they say,

'My friend did it and they were successful', or 'I read a magazine article …' They always want to tell you the bright side. Nobody ever talks about what happens if it never is successful.

Changing clinics

It can be tempting to blame your clinic if your IVF doesn't work, and patients who've had a number of treatment cycles have often been to more than one clinic. The clinics do have varying success rates, and some have more experience at dealing with specific fertility problems than others, but that doesn't mean that you would necessarily have a greater chance of getting pregnant if you change clinic.

Obviously no one would advise staying at a clinic if you didn't feel happy or confident that you were getting good treatment, but there are some advantages to staying put. Your treatment may not have been successful, but doctors will have observed how your body responded, and this is useful when it comes to planning another cycle. You will be familiar with the staff and the way they work, and this may help you feel more relaxed when you start again. If you move to a new clinic, although you can take your medical notes, you may still find that they will want to repeat some tests or to carry out additional ones, and this can feel as if it is slowing the process down.

Helping yourself

This may be a good time to see the clinic counsellor if you haven't already. It can be useful after an unsuccessful cycle to have someone you can talk things through with. Support groups or Internet forums may help, although you will probably feel very raw and sensitive, and if you've made friends with others who are going through treatment at the same time, you may want to avoid the online forums for a while. Having to deal with other people who may have just discovered they are pregnant is not going to be easy.

You may want to consider seeing a complementary therapist after you have had an unsuccessful cycle. They have time to listen, and their treatment may be calming at a time when you are feeling distraught, as this practitioner explains:

> Everybody is always looking at IVF successes, and I think it has to be a lot clearer that it doesn't always work. There's a lot of focus on what doctors are doing, and then suddenly people are left – not having got pregnant – and they need something else to help them. They need something outside that whole process.

Giving up on treatment

Making a decision not to have any more fertility treatment can be extremely difficult. Sometimes people stop because they can't afford to pay for any more IVF, but it can be hard to know when to draw the line if that isn't the main factor in your decision. There is always another clinic to try, another slightly different technique and another consultant holding out the possibility of success.

Doctors sometimes advise patients to stop when there is medical evidence that further cycles are unlikely to succeed, but even if this happens, you will probably be able to find another consultant who is willing to take you on and may suggest trying something slightly different. One of the consultants I spoke to admitted that it can be hard to tell people they ought not to carry on: 'Unfortunately, IVF has become a big business, and lots of couples I see have had numerous treatments. You have to be honest, and I say to them, perhaps it's not to be.'

If you've been producing lots of eggs and good-quality embryos, but not ever getting past the implantation stage, it can be hard to make the decision to give up. Neither doctors nor scientists entirely understand why some embryos don't implant. Annabel has had five unsuccessful IVF cycles, and is saving to pay for a sixth. She says the fact that no one has any idea why her treatment doesn't work has made it difficult to even consider admitting defeat:

> I don't know how many times they've told me the embryos look really good. It gives you so much hope when everything is going well, and when it fails you crash down to earth. At least if things didn't go well you could draw the line and say enough is enough, but when everything goes so well, you just think, *why?*

Some people start out with a definite plan of how many cycles they will do before they give up, but that often changes once they start treatment. Even so, it may be a good idea to think about it at the start, and this fertility nurse says this is advice she makes sure to give to her patients, 'I always say to couples, "Think about when you are going to stop. You do not want to do this forever. It's not good for you, for your sanity or your health," but trying to bring some reality into it can be difficult.'

Eventually, many people get to a point where they just know that they've had enough. You may feel you can't put yourselves through it any more, and sense that it has started to dominate your life in a way that you are finding you can no longer cope with. It may be taking a toll on your relationship, your friendships and your social life, not to mention your finances. You may want to get your career back on track, to make plans for the future, and to start enjoying life again.

Sandra had just had her seventh cycle of IVF when we spoke, and had decided it would be her last attempt:

> It is hard to keep picking yourself up and trying again, and I think it has got harder each time, because you do begin to wonder whether it is actually going to work. We did get to the point where we thought, *we really don't want to do this again*, and that was why we said this was definitely the last time. We feel tired now, and I don't think I've got the energy to do it all again.

Once you've actually made the decision to stop, there will inevitably be sadness, but many people are surprised to find that their overwhelming reaction is relief, and that they can draw strength from finally being able to take control of their lives again and to move on. Alison decided to stop IVF after five treatment cycles, and says it has been a time of very mixed emotions:

> There was just a huge sense of relief that we were not doing it again. There are days when I feel distraught and it really upsets me, but we are starting to think about the future. It feels wonderful to be getting my personality back, and I am slowly but surely beginning to socialise again. I am scared that one day it is all going to come crashing in, and I am going to think, *how am I going to live my life without children*, but it hasn't happened yet.

You may decide that you are going to accept living without children of your own, or that you want to look at adoption as an alternative. Whatever decision you make, you will be able to move on from treatment, to put the negative experiences behind you, and to step forwards towards a more positive future.

Chapter fifteen

A Positive Pregnancy Test – Success at Last

There can be little to match the elation of finally having a positive pregnancy test after all the time and effort of getting there through IVF, and it is a moment you will never forget. Many of us find it hard to believe at first, and I was absolutely convinced the home testing kit I'd used must be faulty when it showed a positive result. Other women have told me that they've tried half a dozen tests before they've finally had to concede that maybe they really are pregnant. By the time we get to this point, most of us have got very used to not being pregnant, to dealing with negative test results and disappointment, and this is uncharted territory. For many couples, a positive pregnancy test is the start of a new journey, but when you've had IVF, it feels more like the end of a particularly long and arduous journey.

The first few weeks

I'd often imagined how wonderful it would be to be pregnant, and had thought that if it ever finally happened, life would be full of nothing but joy and happiness. I hadn't anticipated that pregnancy would bring a whole host of new worries and the elation was soon followed by fears about all the things that could possibly go wrong.

Not everyone feels this way. There are people who get pregnant after IVF who remain perfectly calm and laid-back about the whole thing, who sail through pregnancy relatively easily and refuse to dwell on any potential problems. This is perhaps more likely to be the case among those who get pregnant after their first IVF cycle, and most of us remain very aware of how long it has taken us to get to this point, and worry that if something goes wrong we may never make it this far again.

Scans

One of the nice things about having an IVF pregnancy is that you get to see your baby at such an early stage. You will usually be asked to go back to the fertility clinic a couple of weeks after your pregnancy test for a scan, and I remember ticking off the days as we waited for this. When you've been used to such regular visits to see the doctor or nurse to check on your follicles, a wait of two weeks to check on your baby feels like a lifetime.

You will be able to get your first look at the baby during the scan, and although it is little more than a blob on the ultrasound monitor, you may be able to see the heart beating. It seemed incredible to me that in just a few weeks the tiny embryo had grown into this pulsating little being, and the scan should help you feel more confident about the pregnancy. You may have a second scan at the fertility clinic, but after this most clinics will pass you over to the local maternity service.

The fear of miscarriage

The risk of miscarriage is slightly greater among women who have had IVF than those who have conceived naturally, but you shouldn't dwell on this because it probably has far more to do with other factors than with the treatment itself. We know that women with certain fertility problems are more at risk anyway, as are older women, and the fact that you know you are pregnant so early when you've had IVF explains some of the increase, as women who get pregnant naturally may not always realise if they have a very early miscarriage.

There is no point in spending all your pregnancy worrying about this, although many women find it difficult not to. Isobel's joy at discovering she was pregnant with twins was soon replaced by the fear of miscarriage, and she admits that it plagued her entire pregnancy:

> I was convinced from the start that just because I was pregnant, it didn't necessarily mean I was going to get a baby at the end of it. When I found out it was twins, I was glad because I thought it gave us a better chance that we might lose only one. I was so negative about it, so terrified of bonding with them and then losing them. I just switched off from it, and kept myself believing it wasn't real.

I know it's easier said than done, but as someone who spent most of two IVF pregnancies worrying about things, in retrospect I wish I'd allowed myself to enjoy the experience more, and to worry less. If you are trying to lead a healthy lifestyle, taking your folic acid and being careful about what you eat and drink, you are giving your baby the best possible chance, and you should try to enjoy being pregnant at last.

Just another pregnant woman

Once you've had your final appointments at the fertility clinic, and are under the care of the local maternity service, there may be long gaps between appointments. You will have an initial meeting with a doctor and/or midwife, but after that you may not see anyone for weeks on end. This can be alarming for anyone who is used to the regular monitoring of IVF, but if there were signs of any kind of problem you would be seen more frequently.

If you're worried about something, don't feel afraid to ask. You may feel you are being neurotic, or that you are worried about something silly, but midwives are used to the niggling concerns that women have during pregnancy and will be able to give advice or reassure you. Women who have had IVF do sometimes feel that their entire experience of pregnancy is tainted by worry, as Helena explains:

I felt really tense the whole way through. I remember looking at other people telling people they were pregnant really early and I was thinking, *how do you know that everything is going to be all right?* You are robbed of that joy. Obviously you are happy, but every scan is a real stress.

Pregnancy isn't always easy

The reality of pregnancy can come as a shock when you've spent years imagining how great it will be. Every pregnancy is different, but you may get very sick and tired, and however much you think you'll relish these things as part of pregnancy, it can become overwhelming. Isobel had a particularly difficult pregnancy, and hadn't ever imagined it would be that way:

> I started my morning sickness just a week after embryo transfer, and then I started bleeding. The bleeding carried on until 21 weeks, and I was vomiting eight to ten times a day. I was hospitalised for sickness and bleeding. I was stuck in bed all the time, having expected to be really happy about being pregnant and to have a wonderful time, and the reality was nothing like that at all.

Women who've taken a long time to get pregnant often feel that they can't complain once they've got what they have wanted for so long. Those who've conceived naturally may moan about everything all the way through their pregnancies, but if you've had to have IVF, you may not want to admit to feeling less than marvellous. Sometimes, the doubts and fears can be more fundamental, as this fertility nurse explains:

> There's this holy grail that people are aspiring to because they've lost control over their lives because of the infertility. They don't really think, *do I want to do it?* Then when they get pregnant, like anyone who gets pregnant, they have doubts and wonder whether they want their

lives to change forever, to never have any money and not have any sleep for five to ten years. That gets sidelined when you can't achieve the positive pregnancy test.

Multiple pregnancy

A relatively high percentage of IVF pregnancies are still multiples, and although triplet pregnancies after fertility treatment have thankfully become rare, there are still many IVF twin pregnancies. Carrying twins does make the pregnancy more risky for both mother and babies, and you will be monitored more regularly.

Women who are carrying more than one baby can go into labour early, and are usually booked in to deliver in a hospital that has facilities to care for premature babies in case they need extra medical care. There is a higher Caesarean rate with twins, but many women do give birth to twins naturally. Doctors will make a recommendation about this based on how things have progressed up to this point, and how the babies are positioned.

Birth

Once you get to the point of giving birth, there is no reason this should be different from any other delivery unless there are specific problems that have been identified in advance, or you are carrying twins or triplets. There is sometimes a tendency to categorise an IVF birth as high risk but this shouldn't be the case, if the pregnancy has progressed normally.

You should be guided by your midwife and doctor when you are making decisions about the birth, and shouldn't feel railroaded into plans you aren't happy about just because you've had IVF.

Parenting

Apparently, women who've had IVF babies have an increased risk of getting post-natal depression, and it's easy to see why this could happen. We build our expectations of parenthood so high, both in terms of what it will bring to us, and of what we should be able to give as parents. We imagine we should go through the early years in a blissful haze of domesticity, when in fact the reality of sleepless nights, endless nappy changing and crying babies is tough for anyone. We think we have to find life with a small baby idyllic, and we are often quicker to criticise our own efforts than many other parents. We want to be the perfect parents, always. We don't think we should ever get cross, or tired or irritable. We shouldn't ever snap at our children, or shout. Instead, we should always be at hand with a selection of healthy home-made snacks and a cheery smile.

The pressure can be particularly acute for women who give birth to twins, which is going to be chaotic and exhausting at the best of times. We have to learn to accept that it is not always going to be easy, and that there is nothing wrong with admitting that. Debbie confesses that she found looking after a small baby was far harder than she'd expected: 'I don't know if it is because I'd built up my expectations, but I found it very hard. You do feel you can't complain because you think that people will think, *you wanted this so much, so don't complain about it.'*

We may worry a lot more, too. I remember constantly checking that my son was still breathing when he was tiny, resting my hand on his chest to reassure myself that it was rising and falling normally. I would turn the baby monitor up to peak level when I put him to bed so that I could hear every snuffle, and was forever rolling glasses over the smallest red blemishes on his skin to ensure he didn't have meningitis.

It's hard to believe that, after waiting so long, you finally have what you've always wanted, and that it isn't about to be taken away from you. Even now, 12 years down the line, I still feel lucky to have my children. I may be more relaxed about my unsuccessful attempts to become the perfect mother, but I know how fortunate we were that IVF worked for us. Our children love hearing about how much we wanted them, how we had to get a doctor to help us have them, and how amazed and delighted we were when they were born. They've always been proud of the fact that they were IVF babies because they think it's a very special thing to be. And they're right. There may be more than three million of them worldwide, but an IVF baby is always a truly precious baby.

Appendix

A Brief History of IVF

On top of an office cupboard in a Cambridgeshire fertility clinic sits a rather antiquated glass bell jar. It doesn't look remarkable, but history was made inside it. More than 30 years ago, the world's first IVF baby spent the hours after her conception in a dish inside this very jar. Louise Brown's birth in 1978 heralded a sea change in the hopes and expectations of couples with fertility problems.

Scientists and doctors across the world had been trying to fertilise eggs outside the body for years before Louise Brown was born. They used rabbits for some of the early experiments, and way back in the late nineteenth century embryos had been transferred from one rabbit to another. It wasn't until 1959 that rabbit eggs were successfully fertilised in the laboratory, the first ever *in vitro* fertilisation.

Across the world, teams of scientists and doctors were soon experimenting with human eggs and sperm. Robert Edwards, a scientist based in Cambridge, was fascinated by the idea of fertilising eggs in the laboratory, and the implications this could have for couples who couldn't conceive. His research using human eggs was condemned by many other scientists at the time. They thought it was simply impossible to fertilise a human egg outside the body, and many were worried that if Edwards did eventually succeed, he would end up creating some kind of monster.

If he was to make *in vitro* fertilisation work, Robert Edwards had to find a way of collecting eggs from the ovaries, and he came across a gynaecologist, Patrick Steptoe, who was using a new kind of surgery. Until then, the only way to get access to a woman's womb and ovaries was by cutting right through the abdomen, but Patrick Steptoe had started using a tiny telescope (a laparoscope) which could be inserted through one small cut to get a view of the internal organs. This was known as laparoscopy, and is still used by gynaecologists today. Robert Edwards realised laparoscopy could be the key to collecting eggs from the ovaries, and he began working with Patrick Steptoe in the 1960s.

Although their research progressed in leaps and bounds, they were widely condemned in the media, and by other scientists, for experiments that were considered to be morally wrong. The Medical Research Council refused to give them any funding, and they ended up working in a small cottage hospital, where Patrick Steptoe had to pay for some of their equipment from his own pocket.

Despite all the opposition, women with fertility problems were keen to be involved in their work in the hope that they might be able to conceive against the odds. In 1975, one of the women had the first positive pregnancy test. Much to everyone's dismay, the pregnancy was ectopic and the embryo had implanted in the fallopian tube, so there was no first IVF baby. The lack of belief in their work and the suspicion they faced is epitomised by their experiences when they offered to write about this incredible breakthrough for a medical journal. The editor replied that he could 'see nothing new' in this, the first ever pregnancy from a human egg fertilised in the laboratory.

Edwards and Steptoe had been using drugs to stimulate the ovaries of their female patients, but they realised this wasn't working properly, and so they decided to try IVF in a natural cycle, although this meant there would be only one egg for them to attempt to fertilise. The natural method seemed to work better despite the fact that they didn't have as many eggs, and another patient, Lesley Brown, became pregnant. She went on to give birth to her daughter Louise, the world's first IVF baby, in July 1978.

The bell jar that was home to an embryonic Louise is now kept at Bourn Hall, a private clinic near Cambridge, where Steptoe and Edwards set up the world's first specialist IVF unit. Although they were great pioneers who had achieved a ground-breaking medical advance, even after Louise Brown's birth they were still regarded with suspicion and faced criticism from not just the public and the media but also their fellow medics and scientists. They couldn't get funding to set up a clinic in Cambridge, so they decided to start their own private IVF unit at Bourn.

In the early days, that first specialist IVF centre was a far cry from the comfortable surroundings that we might expect from a private clinic nowadays. The patients who had come from around the world to try this amazing new treatment were housed in a selection of temporary cabins in the grounds. There was still uncertainty about the ethics and morality of creating life in the laboratory, and the work going on at the clinic was viewed as experimental. People questioned the ethics of IVF, and there were concerns that children born that way might have problems later in life, or might be ostracised.

Vivien was thrilled when she was offered a job as a receptionist at the Bourn clinic, having seen reports about IVF on the television. She soon found that not everyone was supportive of her decision to take the job:

It was all very new, and it was amazing. I was proud to be part of that, but people questioned why you would want to work in such a place. At the time it was very controversial and people were really quite short-sighted about it. I think they thought we were playing God.

It wasn't only the staff who had a hard time in the early days, the process was far more complex and demanding for their patients, too. It wasn't something a woman could fit around her normal schedule, as she had to spend days as a hospital inpatient when she had IVF. Relatively, it was far more expensive in those days, costing nearly two thousand pounds for each treatment cycle in the early 1980s. IVF was not widely available, and although other doctors were following in the footsteps of Edwards and Steptoe, there were still only a handful of centres in the world offering the new technique.

The treatment itself was far more invasive, and many of the procedures were complicated. Women had to collect all their urine during the treatment, as this was the only way doctors could monitor their hormone levels. It wasn't so bad doing this if you were an inpatient at the clinic, but it was not so easy during the rest of the treatment, as Judy, who was a patient in those early days, explains:

> I remember carrying this massive container around with me. It was a big plastic canister, see-through so that you could see all this yellow liquid in it. You had to take it to work, or wherever you were, and you had to collect all your urine. Then at the end of the day you had to fill a little bottle for testing, and then you would start again in the morning.

Initially, most IVF was carried out in natural cycles, and doctors had to wait for the hormonal surge that marked ovulation, so they were on call 24 hours a day to carry out egg collection as and when it was necessary. Women had to have a general anaesthetic for egg collection, as this was carried out by laparoscopy and was a far more complex procedure.

The process of transferring the embryos to the womb was very undignified, too. It was believed it would increase the chances of pregnancy if the woman crouched forwards with her chest resting on her knees during embryo transfer. The worst part was that you were expected to stay in the same position for some time afterwards, as Judy recalls: 'They put you in a bed that was cranked up slightly, so that you were facing downhill. I remember I had a cold and a cough, and it was really awkward lying face down. You had to stay like that for at least an hour or maybe two.'

It wasn't just the medical procedures that were different. Emotionally, there was a huge stigma attached to infertility and treatment. If a couple were having problems getting pregnant, it was assumed that something must be wrong with the woman, and doctors didn't always see the male partner at all at first. Perhaps it is not surprising that when couples needed IVF, the men had as little as possible to do with the process. Vivien, who was the receptionist at that first IVF clinic, explains:

> It was so different. Now couples come in and it is a joint thing, they are both going through treatment. Then, it seemed that the woman was having treatment, and the husbands would leave them there. They couldn't stay and there were visiting times for men. It was more of a private thing, too. They didn't want anyone to know because it was all so controversial, and so hush-hush.

The fact that the treatment was still controversial is highlighted by a note about publicity in the information given to patients at the time, which advises them not to communicate in any way with the media and even suggests that they should 'beware of telephone enquiries', taking care not to mention the names of any other patients they'd encountered at the clinic. This attitude is understandable given the media scrum when news of Lesley Brown's pregnancy had leaked out. Journalists were desperately attempting to find out any information they could, and offered thousands of pounds for details about Lesley Brown, or any other women who had been treated at the clinic and might possibly be pregnant.

Despite all the opposition, it wasn't long before more pregnancies followed. Doctors and scientists in other countries had been experimenting in the field at the same time as Edwards and Steptoe, and soon an IVF baby had been born in India, and then in Australia. It was becoming clear that this was not some one-off scientific experiment, but a huge step forward that would change the world for infertile couples.

Scientists and doctors were soon able to freeze spare embryos created during treatment. The first baby was born from a frozen embryo in the 1980s and it seemed one step further down the road to a brave new world. Judy's daughter was an early frozen embryo success, and she remembers staff at the clinic setting her mind at rest about the safety of what they were doing: 'We were told she was the tenth frozen embryo at the clinic. It was exciting to feel that it was all so new, and they reassured me that once the embryo was established there was no reason to suspect that there would be any ill effects from the freezing.'

Doctors began to experiment with different methods of assisted conception. Egg donation, first performed successfully in the 1980s, was a huge breakthrough for women who could not produce their own eggs. The next landmark development came in the early 1990s when scientists managed to fertilise eggs successfully by injecting sperm straight into them. Intra-cytoplasmic sperm injection, or ICSI, gave many more men with fertility problems the chance to father their own genetic children.

In his early days in the laboratory, the IVF pioneer Robert Edwards had realised that it was possible to take one cell out of an embryo without any lasting damage, and developments in this area have allowed couples who have inherited conditions to test embryos to ensure they are healthy.

Meanwhile, ovary transplants and egg and ovarian tissue freezing are being developed as methods of putting female fertility on ice. Egg and ovarian tissue freezing are currently most often used by women who have cancer, as their treatment can leave them infertile. A growing minority are choosing this option for social reasons, and although it's far from a guaranteed way of ensuring you will be able to have a child in the future, it can provide hope for those without any other options, and success rates are improving rapidly.

While some scientists work to improve fertility treatments, others are taking experiments in reproductive technology in different directions. The first successful attempt at cloning resulted in the birth of Dolly the sheep in 1997, and led to questions as to whether human cloning might be just around the corner. Others are working to help cure medical conditions, using hybrid embryos, which were greeted with much controversy, strangely reminiscent of the fears and suspicion that Robert Edwards and Patrick Steptoe faced back in the 1970s, with condemnation that we were on a slippery slope that would inevitably lead to the creation of some kind of half-human monster. Louise Brown, that first baby, has calmly endured the media spotlight over the years, and is now a mother herself, having conceived naturally.

IVF is still young, and there will be many more advances in reproductive technology that will change the face of fertility treatment in the future, but looking back it is quite extraordinary how far we have come in such a relatively short period of time, and we have the perseverance of two men in the face of criticism and ridicule to thank for that.

Resources

International
....

European Society of Human Reproduction and Embryology
www.eshre.com

Fertility Europe
www.fertilityeurope.eu
Association of European organisations offering support
to those who need help to conceive

International Federation of Fertility Societies
www.iffs-reproduction.org

International Premature Ovarian Failure Association
www.pofsupport.org

Australia

Access
www.access.org.au
National infertility support network

Aussie Egg Donors
www.aussieeggdonors.com
Support and information for egg donors and recipients

Australian Acupuncture and Chinese Medicine Association
www.acupuncture.org.au

Australian Homeopathic Association
www.homeopathyoz.org

Australian Multiple Birth Association
www.amba.org.au
Support for families with twins, triplets or more

Donor Conception Support Group of Australia
www.dcsg.org.au

Fertility Society of Australia
www.fertilitysociety.com.au
Represents all those involved in reproductive medicine, as well as providing information for patients

National Institute of Complementary Medicine
www.nicm.edu.au

Polycystic Ovarian Syndrome Association of Australia

www.posaa.asn.au

Support network providing information and advice about polycystic ovary syndrome

Reflexology Association of Australia

www.reflexology.org.au

Ireland

Federation of Irish Complementary Therapy Associations

www.ficta.com

National Infertility Support and Information Group

www.nisig.ie

New Zealand

Advisory Committee on Assisted Reproductive Technology

www.acart.health.govt.nz

Independent advisory committee that formulates advice and guidelines for the regulation of reproductive technology

Fertility NZ

www.fertilitynz.org.nz

Offers information, support and advocacy to those affected by infertility

Inter Country Adoption New Zealand

www.icanz.gen.nz

Inter country adoption agency

Miscarriage Support

www.miscarriagesupport.org.nz

Information and support for those affected by miscarriage

New Zealand Charter of Health Practitioners

www.healthcharter.org.nz

New Zealand Early Menopause Support Group

www.earlymenopause.org.nz

New Zealand Endometriosis Foundation

www.nzendo.co.nz

Support, information and education about endometriosis

New Zealand Homeopathic Society

www.homeopathy.ac.nz

Reflexology New Zealand

www.reflexology.org.nz

Twin Loss NZ

www.twinloss.org.nz

Support group for those who have lost one or more of their children after a multiple pregnancy

South Africa

Homeopathic Association of South Africa
www.hsa.org.za

National Acupuncture and Chinese Medicine Association of South Africa
www.nacmasa.co.za

South African Menopause Society
www.menopause.co.za

South African Reflexology Society
www.sareflexology.org.za

South African Society of Obstetricians and Gynaecologists
www.sasog.co.za

United Kingdom

ACeBabes
www.acebabes.co.uk
Support for those who are expecting a baby, or who have become parents, after fertility treatment

Aromatherapy Council
www.aromatherapycouncil.co.uk

Association of Clinical Embryologists
www.embryologists.org.uk

Association of Reflexologists
www.aor.org.uk

Adoption UK
www.adoptionuk.org
Support for adoptive families before, during and after adoption

British Association for Adoption and Fostering
www.baaf.org.uk

British Fertility Society
www.fertility.org.uk
Represents professionals working in reproductive medicine

British Infertility Counselling Association
www.bica.net
Information on fertility counselling, including help in finding a counsellor

CHANA
www.chana.org.uk
Support network for Jewish couples with fertility problems

Daisy Network
www.daisynetwork.org.uk

Charity offering support and information for women who have experienced a premature menopause

Donor Conception Network

www.dcnetwork.org
Self-help network for families created with the help of donor gametes, those seeking to start a family this way and adults conceived using a donor

Endometriosis SHE trust

www.shetrust.org.uk

Endometriosis UK

www.endometriosis-uk.org
Information and support for women living with endometriosis

Fertile Hope

www.fertilehope.org
Support for cancer patients facing infertility

General Hypnotherapy Register

www.general-hypnotherapy-register.com

Human Fertilisation and Embryology Authority

www.hfea.gov.uk
Regulates UK fertility clinics, and gives information on the clinics and their success rates

Infertility Network UK

www.infertilitynetworkuk.com
National charity offering information, support and advice

Institute for Complementary and Natural Medicine
www.i-c-m.org.uk

The Miscarriage Association
www.miscarriageassociation.org.uk
Support and information for those suffering the effects
of pregnancy loss

More To Life
www.moretolife.co.uk
Support for the involuntarily childless

Mothers 35 plus
www.mothers35plus.co.uk
Information, support and advice for older mothers

Multiple Births Foundation
www.multiplebirths.org.uk
Charity providing information, education and support

National Gamete Donation Trust
www.ngdt.co.uk
Provides information about egg and sperm donation

Oasis
www.adoptionoverseas.org
Overseas adoption support and information service

Pink Parents
www.pinkparents.org.uk
Support for lesbian and gay parents

Progress Educational Trust

www.progress.org.uk

Information and debate on assisted reproduction and human genetics

The Reiki Association

www.reikiassociation.org.uk

Royal College of Obstetricians and Gynaecologists

www.rcog.org.uk

Society of Homeopaths

www.homeopathy-soh.org

Surrogacy UK

www.surrogacyuk.org

Support and information for anyone with an interest in surrogacy

TAMBA

www.tamba.org.uk

Twins and Multiple Births Association

Verity

www.verity-pcos.org.uk

Support and information for women affected by polycystic ovary syndrome

United States of America

American Fertility Association
www.theafa.org
Provides information about infertility and treatment

American Society for Reproductive Medicine
www.asrm.org
Organisation devoted to advancing knowledge about infertility and reproductive medicine

Early Menopause
www.earlymenopause.com
Information, advice and discussion

National Center for Homeopathy
www.nationalcenterforhomeopathy.org

The Endometriosis Association
www.endometriosisassn.org

Reflexology Association of America
www.reflexology-usa.org

Resolve – The National Infertility Association
www.resolve.org
Offers support and information

Recommended Reading

Black, Rachel and Seull, Louise, *Beyond Childlessness*, Rodale, 2005

McGuckin, Isla, *Pink for a Girl*, Hay House, 2006

Glossary

Blastocyst: An embryo which has been developing for about five days since conception.

Cervix: The entrance to the womb from the vagina.

Chlamydia: A sexually transmitted infection which can cause fertility problems.

Down-regulating drugs: These drugs are often prescribed at the start of an IVF cycle to switch off your hormonal cycle.

Ectopic pregnancy: An ectopic pregnancy occurs when an egg implants outside the womb, usually in the fallopian tube. It will not lead to a viable pregnancy.

Embryo: A fertilised egg.

Endometriosis: A condition where tissue similar to the womb lining grows outside the womb.

Endometrium: The lining of the womb which grows during each menstrual cycle and is shed during the period.

Fallopian tubes: The tubes which lead from each ovary to the womb.

Fibroid: A benign growth found in or around the womb.

Follicle-stimulating hormone (FSH): A hormone that stimulates the ovary to produce follicles.

Gamete: A sperm or egg.

Gonadotrophins: Drugs used to stimulate the ovaries.

ICSI (Intra-cytoplasmic sperm injection): A variation of IVF during which sperm is injected into the egg to try to fertilise it.

IVM (In vitro maturation): IVM involves taking eggs direct from the ovary when they are still immature, and developing them in the laboratory ready for fertilisation.

Laparoscopy: An examination of the reproductive organs using a tiny telescope which is inserted into the abdomen.

Mild or soft IVF: Mild IVF uses lower doses of drugs so the ovaries do not produce as many eggs, causing less disruption to the woman's body.

Oestrogen: Hormone produced by the ovary.

Ovarian Hyperstimulation Syndrome (OHSS): A condition where the ovaries are over-stimulated during fertility treatment which can become serious.

Ovarian reserve: This is the term used for the egg-producing capacity of the ovary which declines with age.

Ovulation: The moment when an egg is released from a follicle in the ovary.

PGD (Pre-implantation genetic diagnosis): PGD is used to screen an embryo for inherited conditions by testing one or two cells.

PGS (Pre-implantation genetic screening): PGS uses a similar process of testing cells to PGD, but it is used to check embryos for chromosomal problems.

Polycystic ovary syndrome (PCOS): A female hormonal problem which may disrupt ovulation and lead to infertility.

Progesterone: Hormone produced after ovulation.

Surrogacy: During a surrogate pregnancy, one woman will agree to carry a child for another woman or couple.

Index

acupuncture 203–6
administration staff 58
adoption 233
age
    and female fertility 13–14,
        64, 224
    and miscarriage risk 224
alcohol intake 121–2, 162–3,
    189–90
AMH (anti-Mullerian hormone)
    64
anaesthetics 89, 94–5
andrologists 57
aneuploidy screening *see* PGS
antral follicle count 64, 65
anxieties
    calming your 213
    during pregnancy 235, 236–9
aromatherapy 209
aspirin 82–3
assessing your need for IVF
    15–25
assisted hatching 45–6
attitude 143–4, 197

Bach flower remedies 213–14
bed rest 116–17
biological clock 3, 13–14, 167
birth 239–40
blastocysts 104–5, 109
bleeding
    during pregnancy 123–4,
        238
    implantation 124
bloating 80, 85
blood tests 64, 80–1
Body Mass Index (BMI) 30,
    192–3
Bourn Hall 244–6
Brown, Lesley 244, 247
Brown, Louise 242, 244, 250

caffeine 193
calming treatments 204, 209
    see also relaxation
cancelled cycles 86
cannabis 191
capacitation 9
centrifuges 97–8
cervix 66, 112

CHILD 2
chlamydia 12–13, 65
clinics
    atmosphere 30–1
    changing 59, 229
    checklist 36
    choosing 26–46
    consulting rooms 5
    costs 29
    counselling rooms 53
    eligibility status 29–30
    first appointments 58–60
    history of 244–6
    laboratories 52–3
    lesbian couples and 34–5
    location 31–2
    men and 163–5
    men's rooms 51–2, 88
    operating theatres 52
    as part of larger hospitals
        48
    personal recommendations
        regarding 35–6
    recovery rooms 94–5
    reputations 35–6
    satellite 32–3
    single women and 34–5
    size of 48–9
    specialisms 30
    staff 53–8
    success rates 28
    support 33–4, 38
    transport units 33
    and treatment 29–30
    and types of treatment 40–6
    visiting 27
    waiting rooms 49–51
    waiting times 28
    see also overseas clinics
cloning 249–50

CMV-status testing 65
communication skills 138
complementary therapies
        18–19, 198, 201–19, 230
    caution regarding 216–17
    costs of 218–19
    directory 203–16
    men and 218
confidentiality issues 150–1
consent issues 70
consultants 54–5
consulting rooms 5
control, loss of 128–30
costs 29, 80, 143–4
    see also discount treatments
counselling 33–4, 120, 145–56,
        174
    confidentiality issues
        150–1
    crisis points 152–3
    for donor gamete use 154–5,
        179–82
    for failed treatments 225,
        230
    implications 146
    men and 154, 170–1
    for miscarriage 225
    opting out of 155–6
    post-treatment 153–4
    process 148–52
    support 146
    and surrogacy 154–5,
        179–82
    therapeutic 146–7
    timing 151–2
counselling rooms 53
counsellors 53, 147–8, 180–1
craniosacral therapy 213
crisis counselling 152–3
culture mediums 95

cumulus cells 95–6
cycles (IVF) 6

defining IVF 5–6, 40
delivery 239–40
denial 23–4
depression 127–8
  post-natal 240
diet, healthy 122, 162–3, 193
disclosure, regarding donor
  gamete use to kids 181–2
discount treatments 176–7
doctors 54–5, 202
donor eggs 37–8, 64, 172,
  174–8, 248
  and counselling 154–5,
  179–82
  from abroad 185–6
  known-donors 175
  support for the use of 186–7
donor sperm 37–8, 161–2,
  172–4, 178–87
  and counselling 154–5,
  179–82
  from abroad 172–3, 185–6
  known-donors 174
  and lesbian couples 185
  and single women 183–4
  support for the use of 186–7
down-regulation 68, 77, 78–9,
  166
drugs, recreational 191
drugs regimes 6, 16, 42, 68,
  77–84
  down-regulation 68, 77,
  78–9, 166
  hCG (human chorionic
  gonadotrophin) injections
  82
  immune therapy 82–4

ovary stimulating drugs 77,
  79–81, 87
  prices 80
  side effects 78–9

eating disorders 11
ectopic pregnancy 221, 226–7
Edwards, Robert 242–4, 248,
  249
egg collection 33, 87–92
  history of 243, 246
  in the operating theatre 52,
  90–2
  preparing for 89–90
  and semen samples 87–9
  and time off work 72
egg fertilisation
  failure 101–2
  in ICSI 100
  in the lab 98, 101–3
  in natural reproduction
  9–10
egg preparation 77–92
  cancelled cycles 86
  drugs regimes 77–84
  egg collection 87–92
  and ovarian hyperstimulation
  syndrome 84–6
  and soft/mild IVF 86–7
egg-sharing schemes 176–7
eggs
  effects of aging on 64
  embryologists and 56–7
  freezing 52, 57, 249
  and the history of IVF
  242–4
  and the IVF process 6
  lab work on 94, 95–6,
  101–3, 106
  natural production 7–8

see also donor eggs; ovulation (egg production)
embryo transfer 6, 102–3, 109–24
  complementary therapies and 203
  frozen 46, 114–15, 248
  and the history of IVF 246
  and implantation 115
  number of embryos 109–11
  and ovarian hyperstimulation syndrome 85–6
  preparation for 108
  process 111–15
  telling others about 117–18
  and time off work 73, 117
  trial 65–6
  'two-week wait' 115–24
embryologists 56–7, 92, 93–104, 106, 112–13, 115, 160
embryos
  assisted hatching 45–6
  checking for inherited conditions 43–4, 249
  embryologists and 56–7
  fragmentation 103
  freezing 29, 52, 57, 107–8, 111, 248
  grading 103–4
  lab work on 94, 96, 102–4, 106, 108
  and natural reproduction 10
  spare 70
  storage costs 29
  thawing 108
  viewing 53
emotional impact of IVF 81, 118–19, 125–44
  men and 167–8

and secondary infertility 136–7
  self-help for 138–43
  see also feelings towards IVF
endometriosis 12
energy healing 214–15
essential oils 209
expectations 25

failed treatments 220–33
  trying again 227–9
failure, feelings of 130–1
fallopian tubes 8, 9
  and ectopic pregnancy 226–7
  and GIFT/ZIFT 41
  problems with 12–13, 15
families, dealing with 134–5
fears
  calming your 213
  during pregnancy 235, 236–9
feelings towards IVF 19–25
  see also emotional impact of IVF
female factor infertility 10–14, 131
fertilisation *see* egg fertilisation
fertility boosters
  complementary therapies 201–19
  lifestyle changes 188–200
fertility rituals/myths 199–200
fibroids 12, 17, 65
flower remedies 213–14
fluid balance 84
folic acid 19, 122, 194

follicle-stimulating hormone (FSH) 7, 8, 63, 64, 79
follicles 7, 8
  antral follicle count 64, 65
  and egg collection 91
  and ovarian hyperstimulation syndrome 85
  resting 42
  and stimulating drugs 79, 81
friends 135–6, 141–2
FSH *see* follicle-stimulating hormone
full blood count 64

genetic screening 43–4, 249
German measles *see* rubella
GIFT (gamete intra-fallopian transfer) 41
giving up IVF 230–3
gonadotrophins 68
  see also hCG (human chorionic gonadotrophin)

hCG (human chorionic gonadotrophin)
  injections 82
  and ovarian hyperstimulation syndrome 84
  pregnancy tests and 221
healthy lifestyles 19, 188–200
heparin 82–3
hepatitis 29, 62
herbalism 206–7, 217
history of IVF 242–50
HIV 29
  testing for 62
holistic approaches 201, 205, 216
homeopathy 210–11, 218

hormonal problems, female 10, 11–12
hot flushes 78
Human Fertilisation and Embryology Authority 3
hydrosalpinx 13
hypnotherapy 211–13

ICSI (intra-cytoplasmic sperm injection) 89, 248
  defining 40–1
  lab work 95–6, 98–100
  men and 160, 162–6
ICSI rig (micromanipulators) 99
immune therapy 82–4
implantation 115
  bleeding 124
  complementary therapies and 204
  mysteries of 231
  outside the womb 226
  in vitro 6
incubators 100–1
infertility
  female factor 10–14, 131
  male factor 14–15, 130, 158–62
  secondary 14, 136–7
  stigma of 49, 246–7
  unexplained 2–3, 14, 21
Infertility Network UK 3, 140, 142–3, 158, 168
information sources 24–5, 66–8, 138–9, 198
inherited conditions, screening for 43–4, 249
inhibin B 64
injections 68–70, 78, 165–6
insulin 11

Internet
  misinformation on 142–3
  as source of support 24–5,
    34, 67, 141–3, 157
intra-cytoplasmic sperm
  injection *see* ICSI
isolation 126–7, 135, 137
IUI (intrauterine insemination)
  17–18, 21, 160
  using donor sperm 172
IVIg (intravenous immu-
  noglobulin G treatment) 83
IVM (*in vitro* maturation) 42

jealousy 131–2, 176

laboratories 52–3
laboratory stage 92, 93–108
  blastocysts 104–5
  eggs 94, 95–6, 101–3,
    106
  embryos 94, 96, 102–4,
    106, 108
  fertilisation 101–3
  freezing gametes 107–8
  grading embryos 103–4
  ICSI 95–6, 98–100
  incubators 100–1
  sperm 94, 95, 96–100,
    106
  thawing gametes 108
  witnessing 106
laparoscopy 243, 246
lesbian couples 34–5, 172,
  174, 183, 185
Lewis-Jones, Clare 140, 142–3,
  158, 168
LH (luteinising hormone) 8,
  64, 79
lifestyle changes 19, 188–200

living without children 233
loneliness 126–7, 135, 137

medical model 202
medical records 59
meetings, pre-treatment 66–7
men 157–71
  and complementary thera-
    pies 218
  and counselling 154, 170–1
  dealing with other people
    168–9
  and IVF/ICSI cycles 162–6
  male factor infertility 14–15,
    130, 158–62
  physical examinations for 58
  support from 162, 163–7
  and support groups 169–70
  and their emotions 167–8
  treatments for male infer-
    tility 160–2
menopausal symptoms 78–9,
  166
menopause, early/premature 11
men's rooms 51–2, 88
menstrual cycle
  irregular 11
  see also ovulation; periods
meridians 204
MESA (micro-epididymal
  sperm aspiration) 44
midwives 237
miscarriage 223–5
  and complementary thera-
    pies 216–17
  fear of 236–7
  prevention 82, 204
  recurrent 224
Montuschi, Olivia 180, 182,
  186, 187

morning sickness 238
multiple pregnancy 3, 18, 105, 109–11, 239, 240
multivitamins 122, 163, 194
Muslims 22

nasal sprays 78, 79
natural-cycle IVF 41–2
nature, and IVF 22–3
naturopaths 217
need for IVF, assessing your 15–25
neural tube defects 122
night sweats 78
nurses 55–6
nutritional supplements 194
nutritional therapy 215–16

obesity 191–3
oestrodial 64
oestrogen 7–8
operating theatres 52
other people
    dealing with 133–6, 168–9
    telling about IVF 73–6, 117–18, 223
ovarian drilling, laparoscopic 17
ovarian hyperstimulation syndrome (OHSS) 42, 84–6
ovarian reserve testing 63–4, 65
ovarian stimulating drugs 77, 79–81
    and soft/mild IVF 87
ovarian tissue freezing 249
ovaries 7
    problems with 13
overseas clinics 36–9, 122–3
    donor eggs from 185–6

donor sperm from 172–3, 185–6
    and surrogacy 178
overweight 11, 29–30
ovulation (egg production) 7–8, 246
    disruption 10–11
    and intrauterine insemination 17–18

pain relief 89
paperwork 70
parenting 240–1
pelvic inflammatory disease 12
periods
    starting 123–4
    see also menstrual cycle
personality change 131–2
PESA (percutaneous sperm aspiration) 44
PGD (pre-implantation genetic diagnosis) 43
PGS (pre-implantation genetic screening) 43–4
physical examinations
    female 58–9
    male 58
physical exercise 194–5
polar body 95
polycystic ovary syndrome (PCOS) 10–11, 42, 84, 225
positive outlook 143–4
post-natal depression 240
pre-treatment program 61–76
    meetings 66–7
    paperwork 70
    telling others 73–6
    tests 61–6

understanding your
treatment 66–70
and work commitments
70–3
pregnancy 234–40
anxieties during 235, 236–9
bleeding during 123–4, 238
early signs of 119–20
ectopic 221, 226–7
multiple 3, 18, 105, 109–11,
239, 240
reality of 238–9
pregnancy tests 220–2
blood tests 221
home testing 220–1
low positive results 221–2
negative 222–3
positive 234–41
'two-week wait' for 115–24
premature babies 110, 239
progesterone supplements 122
prolactin, raised levels 11–12
pronucleate stage 101

qi 204

receptionists 53–4
recovery rooms 94–5
reflexology 207–9
refusing IVF 20–1
reiki 214–15
relationships 132–6
relaxation 201, 208–9, 211–13,
215, 219
see also calming treatments
religion 22
reproduction 7–10
see also sexual intercourse
Roman Catholicism 22
rubella 62

screening, for inherited conditions 43–4, 249
secondary infertility 14, 136–7
sedation 89–90, 94–5
self-care 198
semen 8, 15, 18
see also sperm
semen analysis 63
semen samples 51, 63
at the egg collection stage
87–9
embarrassment about giving
87–9
poor 89
seminal fluid 8
seminologists 57, 63
sexual intercourse 7, 8–9, 122,
133
see also reproduction
sexually transmitted infections
12–13, 65
shame 130–1
siblings 137
single women 34–5, 172, 174,
183–4
smoking 121, 188–9
soft/mild IVF 42, 86–7
specialisms 30
sperm
absence of 15
embryologists and 56–7
and fertilisation 9–10, 98
freezing 52, 57
grading 96–7
harvesting the best 97–8
and ICSI 40–1, 98–100
and IUI 18
and the IVF process 6
lab work on 94, 95, 96–100,
106

morphology 15
motility 96–7
production 8, 14–15, 162–3
quality 15, 96–7
and sexual intercourse 8–9
surgical retrieval 44–5
swimup procedure 97
washing 97–8
see also donor sperm
sperm antibody test 63
sperm count 14–15, 97, 158–9,
160
tips for improving 162–3
spina bifida 122
staff 53–8
Steptoe, Patrick 243–4, 248
sterilisation, reversal 17, 44,
160–1
steroids 83
anabolic 191
stigma
of infertility 49, 246–7
of IVF 23–4
stimulated cycles 18
stress 117, 195–6
success rates 28
successful treatments 234–41
support 33–4, 38, 75–6, 120,
127–8
for donor gamete use
186–7
from partners 162, 163–7
online 24–5, 34, 67, 141–3,
157
see also counselling
support groups 24, 34, 120,
140–1, 169–70
surgery 17
surgical sperm retrieval 44–5
surrogacy 37, 177–9

counselling for 154–5,
179–82
overseas 178
swimup procedure 97

telling others 73–6, 117–18,
223
TESE (testicular sperm extraction) 44, 45
'test-tube babies' 6
testicles 8, 163
testosterone 8, 11, 159
tests 61–6, 80–1
time, giving yourself 21–2
traditional Chinese medicine 206
see also acupuncture
transport units 33
treatment
assessing your needs for
15–25
breaks from 227–8
discount 176–7
egg preparation 77–92
failed 220–33
the laboratory 93–108
men and 162–6
refusal 20–1
successful 234–41
types 40–6
see also pre-treatment
program
trial embryo transfer 65–6
trying again 227–9
twins 105, 110–11, 239, 240
'two-week wait' 115–24

ultrasound scans 65, 113,
235–6
of the pregnancy 221–2
vaginal 58–9, 81, 90

underweight, severe 193
unexplained infertility 2–3,
    14, 21

vaginal mucus 9
vaginal ultrasound scans 58–9,
    81, 90
vasectomy reversal 17, 44,
    160–1
visualisation techniques 118
vitrification 107–8

waiting rooms 49–51
waiting times 28

weight 191–3
witnessing 106
womb 7, 13
work commitments 129
    and embryo transfer 117
    job stress 117
    and pre-treatment programs
        70–3
worrying 200

yoga 215

ZIFT (zygote intra-fallopian
    transfer) 41

Also by Kate Brian

The Complete Guide to Female Fertility

ISBN 978 0 7499 2792 9

With warnings about rising infertility rates and the dangers of leaving motherhood too late, many women are concerned about when or whether they will manage to have a baby. At the same time, news of the latest advances in reproductive technology suggests it may be possible to beat the female biological clock and put childbearing on hold.

Kate Brian is an expert on fertility and *The Complete Guide to Female Fertility* is a practical and accessible guide which addresses all the questions women have about their fertility and getting pregnant. It deals with the medical facts, the emotions and the social aspects of female fertility, and includes the real-life experiences and insights of dozens of women.

The Complete Guide to Female Fertility gives the facts in a balanced, down-to-earth manner and includes information on:

- how your reproductive system works
- when you are at your most fertile
- how your age affects your chances of conceiving
- how you can boost your fertility naturally
- what may stop you getting pregnant
- what reproductive technology can do to help.